A Simple and
Clarity, Purpos

CREATING
VIBRANT HEALTH

by

Douglas Lobay, N.D.

**A Practical Roadmap to Enlightenment, Inner
Peace and Optimal Health.**

Canadian Cataloguing in Publication Data
Lobay, Doug 1965-

Includes Index
ISBN: 0-9695861-2-6

1. Naturopathy - Handbooks, manuals, etc... 2. Natural Health 3. Psychology
I. Title

Published by
Apple Communications
Kelowna, B.C.

Printed in Canada

Acknowledgements

I would like to thank:

Mom and Dad
Arlene and Jim
Mike and Annette
Mike and Nellie
Dr. Gaetano Morello
Dr. Garrett Swetlikoff
Dr. Kim Vanderlinden
Susan Carroll
Natalie, Rachel and Jessica

Dedication

To Rachel and Jessica
For all their love, guidance and support

Table Of Contents

> It's not only important to
> add years to your life, but to
> add life to your years.

Quotations

"A musician must make music, an artist must paint, a poet must write, if he is to be ultimately at peace with himself."

Abraham Maslow

"People measure their esteem of each other by what each has, and not by what each is...Nothing can bring you peace but yourself."

Ralph Waldo Emerson

"No where can a man find a quieter or more untroubled retreat than his own soul."

Marus Aurelius

Introduction

I was originally going to title this book "My Personal Tibet." I mentioned this title to a dozen patients and half the patients didn't get it and didn't like it. So in the name of good marketing I decided to call this book "Creating Vibrant Health." This title is pro-active and uplifting. It is meant that the patient or individual takes responsibility and the initiative for creating and developing their health. It is a simple and practical guide to achieving clarity, purpose, enlightenment and inner peace in every day life. I've written about the importance of diet and good health and the value of nutritional supplementation. Now I've come full circle and have written a book on the importance of your mental, emotional and spiritual health.

"Creating Vibrant Health" is a lot like searching for your own spiritual Tibet. I've always dreamed about going to Tibet, but I've never been there. In fact, this book really isn't about Tibet at all. Rather this book is about what Tibet represents. Growing up in a small town I've always fantasized about travelling to exotic places, visiting unique cultures and meeting different people. I hope that in my life time I afford the opportunity to actually physically visit Tibet and sample its unique culture. To me, Tibet embodies a far off mystical place with a radically different culture and distinctly different people. Tibet is shrouded in mystery and intrigue. It is geographically located on the other side of the world in Asia. Tibet includes one the largest and tallest mountain ranges in the world, the Himalayans. It borders Mount Everest, the tallest mountain in the world. The grandeur and vastness of these mountains is awesome. The snow covered peaks reach up into the sky into the deep universe. They seem to touch the gates of heaven. The glistening mountains reflect the sun and moon light through hazy ethereal circular clouds like the cover of a gospel cd. In between the large mountains are vast, wind swept, desolate plains and lush, fertile valleys. There is a strong sense of reverence and sacred beauty about the Himalayans and Tibet. It would be a spiritually enlightening experience visiting Tibet and these sacred mountains.

As a practicing naturopathic family physician who specializes in preventive and nutritional medicine I see a wide variety of complaints, illness and disease. Many of the symptoms and complaints are physical in nature and our treatment is aimed at improving these. I frequently recommend dietary changes and nutritional supplementation including vitamins, minerals, homeopathic medicines and herbal medicines. While important I always contend that our mental, emotional and spiritual state is as is important and frequently overlooked. I've always stated that you can make tremendous changes in your diet and take good vitamins and minerals, but you must be clear about your mental and spiritual goals. You must be clear about who you are, what you stand for and where you want to go? This is true no matter what your goals in life are. Whether they are materialistic, spiritual or health oriented, you must be clear in what it is you want to achieve.

This book is about achieving positive direction, enlightenment and inner peace in every day life. You don't have to go to Tibet or some other far off and distant place to achieve some clarity in your life. This book is part entertainment, part work book and part thought provoking reflection. The first activity of this book is to clarify your values, attitudes and beliefs. Before you can achieve enlightenment and inner peace you must know what you stand for and what you believe. Next you must be clear on what it is you want in life for yourself or others. Then you must take specific action to achieve what you want and make things happen. You must learn to manage your emotion and learn effective time management and problem solving skills. In our face paced society it is easy to become overwhelmed and stressed out. You must learn to relax and practice natural stress management techniques. You should strive to practice forgiveness and gratitude and live in the present moment. Only then can you take the steps to achieve inner peace and find your self-fulfilling

original but it includes what has influenced me the most. I've tried
to make it simple and easy to understand. Like a romance novel
I've tried to make it engrossing and captivating..

James Hilton wrote the hugely popular book, "The Lost
Horizon" about a group of travellers who stumbled upon a virtual
Shangri-La in a far off and distant land. The book was eventually
made into a feature film about their experiences there.

_"That evening, after dinner, Conway made occasion to
leave the others and stroll out into the calm, moon-washed
courtyards. Shangri-La was lovely then, touched with the mystery
that lies at the core of al loveliness. The air was cold and still; the
mighty spire of Karakal looked nearer, much nearer than by
daylight. Conway was physically happy, emotionally satisfied,
and mentally at ease; but in his intellect, which was not quite the
same thing as mind, there was a little stir...Passing along a
cloister, he reached the terrace leaning over the valley. The scent
of tuberose assailed him, full of delicate associations; in China it
was called "the smell of moonlight." He thought whimsically that
if moonlight has a sound also, it might well be the Rameau gavotte
he had heard so recently; and that set him thinking of the little
Manchu. It has not occurred to him to picture women at Shangri-
La; one did not associate their presence with the general practice
of monasticism."_

_"He gazed over the edge into the blue-black emptiness.
The drop was phantasmal; perhaps as much as a mile. He
wondered if he would be allowed to descend it and inspect the
valley civilization that had been talked of. The notion of this
strange culture-pocket, hidden amongst unknown ranges, and
ruled over by some vague kind of theocracy, interested his as a
student of history, apart form the curious though perhaps related
secrets of the lamasery."_

_"Suddenly on a flutter of air, came sounds from far below.
Listening intently, he could hear gongs and trumpets and also
(though perhaps only in imagination) the massed wail of voices._

The sounds faded on a veer of the wind, then returned to fade again. But the hint of life and liveliness in those veiled depths served only to emphasize the austere serenity of Shangri-La. Its forsaken courts and pale pavilions simmered in repose from which all the fret of existence had ebbed away, leaving a hush af if moments hardly dared to pass. Then, from a window high above the terrace, he caught the rose-gold of lantern light; was it there that the lamas devoted themselves to contemplation and the pursuit of wisdom, and were those devotions now in progress?"

I hope you enjoy this compilation of the many books and people I've come across. I must confess it is not all original. It represents the most poignant and impressionable quotes and information I've come across. I want to make it practical and interactive. Like a computer program I've tried to make it simple and user friendly. I've asked many questions that demand that you think about them and more importantly write the answers in the space provided. Keep on open mind, read it, reflect on it and enjoy it. I hope that it leaves you with a lasting impression of how you can take charge of your life and how you can create vibrant life.

Sincerely,

Doug Lobay

Chapter 1

Values, Attitudes and Beliefs

To begin our journey of achieving inner health you must clarify exactly what your values, attitudes and beliefs are. You must first know who you are and what you stand for? Then you can outline the type of person you want to become by setting goals. Your goals must be in alignment with your values, attitudes and beliefs. Then you can take action towards achieving your goals and becoming the type of person you set for yourself.

All You Need to Know

Robert Fulghum wrote the simple yet profound book, "All I Ever Needed to Know I Learned in Kindergarten." He writes about the real life experiences that we all have at a young age while in preschool and kindergarten. Many of the lessons and wisdom we attain at this young age influences our behavior in adulthood. All the simple truths we learned are true to life at all ages.

"Most of what I really need to know about how to live and what to do and how to be, I learned in kindergarten. Wisdom was not at the top of the graduate mountain, but there in the sandbox at the nursery school."

"These are the things I learned: Share everything. Play fair. Don't hit people. Put things back where you found them. Clean up your own mess. Don't take things that aren't yours. Say you're sorry when you hurt somebody. Wash your hands before

you eat. Flush. Warm cookies and cold milk are good for you. Live a balanced life. Learn some and think some and draw and paint and sing and dance and play and work every day some."

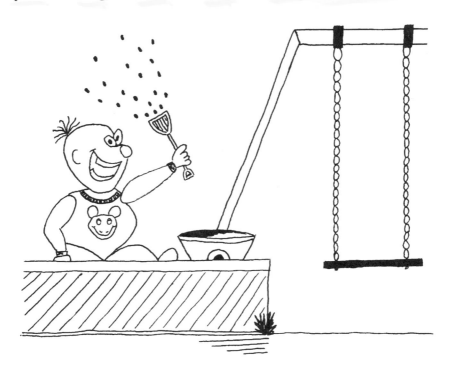

"Take a nap every afternoon. When you go out into the world, watch for traffic, hold hands and stick together. Be aware of wonder. Remember the little seed in the plastic cup. The roots go down and the plant goes up and nobody really knows how or why, but we are all like that."

"Goldfish and hamsters and white mice and even the little seed in the plastic cup -- they all die. So do we."

"And then remember the book about Dick and Jane and the first word you learned, the biggest word of all: LOOK. Everything you need to know is in there somewhere. The Golden Rule and love and basic sanitation. Ecology and politics and sane living."

"Think about what a better world it would be if we all -- the whole world -- had cookies and milk about 3 o'clock every afternoon and then lay down with our blankets for a nap. Or if we had a basic policy in our nations to always put things back where we found them and cleaned up our own messes. And it is still true, no matter how old you are, when you go out into the world, it is better to hold hands and stick together."

Values

What do you value in your life? Do you value life? Do you value yourself? A value is a quality that makes something worth having. It is something that we regard as important and ascribe some worth to. Something we value is considered valuable and highly esteemed. We may value physical, material possessions. We may value our house, automobile, boat, clothes, jewelry, paintings, computer, television, stereo and other physical possessions that have great monetary value. We may value day to day activities, hobbies and leisure activities. But some of the most important things we value close to our heart are non-physical, immaterial and of little or no monetary value. We may value our personal memories and past experiences. This can include a picture or an heirloom that has great personal significance and value, but has little outward, monetary value. A value may be a deeply private and personal principle, belief or custom that is important and valuable to you; right or wrong; good or bad. Some common values include love, god or other higher spiritual being, goals, self, communication, respect, fun, growth, support, challenge, creativity, beauty, activities, freedom and honesty.

Identify what physical and material possessions you value.

1. _____

2. _____

3. _____

4. _____

5. _____

6. _____

7. _____

8. _____

9. _____

10. _____

Next write down non-physical and immaterial things you value. Examine your life and evaluate what you value the most and deepest at your own personal core.

1. _____

2. _____

3. _____

4. _____

5. _____

6. _____

7. _____

8. _____

9. _____

10. _____

Copy: page 80 — 89

Esteemed Value

Esteem means to think highly of; regard as valuable and regard with respect. We often place esteemed value on material and physical possessions. We also place esteemed value on famous people including actors, actresses, politicians, sports figures and other individuals of notoriety. However, we often lack esteemed value on what we should value most, ourselves. Self-esteem means to think highly of yourself; regard yourself as valuable and regard yourself with respect. You must realize that you are unique and special. There is no one else like you among the six billion people on the earth. You have a special place and a unique purpose. You must cultivate your self-worth, develop your self-esteem and strive to develop your full potential. Begin to develop your self-esteem by changing your attitude about yourself.

Attitude

Attitude is a way of feeling or thinking. How you feel or what you think can influence your health and well being. An attitude can be developed by your reaction to the external circumstances around you. An attitude can also be developed by simply changing your thoughts and what your thinking. Since you can control your thoughts and what you think, you can control and change your attitude. Your attitude can be good or bad, positive or negative, healthy or sick. Attitudes are often manifested by our emotions. And since you can change your attitude and outlook, you can change your emotions by thinking and your thoughts.

Victor Frankl and the Nazis

While in college a close friend recommended that I read a remarkable book about a man who was imprisoned in a Nazi concentration camp during World War II. Viktor Frankl wrote the short book, "Man's Search for Meaning" about his experiences there. He does not highlight the unspeakable horrors and atrocities that were common in the concentration camps, but rather focuses on his attitudes and beliefs.

> *"We who lived in the concentration camps can remember men who walked thought the huts comforting others, giving away their last piece of bread. They may have been few in number, but they offer sufficient proof that everything can be taken from a man but one thing: The last of his freedoms--to choose one's attitude in any given set of circumstances, to choose one's own way."*

Attitude Adjustment

To change your attitude you can take steps towards the way you think or feel about some particular process in your life. Think of all the positive benefits of changing your attitude and the negative side effects of maintaining your current attitude.

Write down an attitude that you want to change right now. Why did you experience that old attitude and what a new attitude will mean to you? What are the positive benefits of having this new attitude and how will it make you feel better right now?

_____

_____

_____

_____

_____

_____

_____

Bernie Siegel, Love and Healing

Bernie Siegel is a Connecticut surgeon who has spent his entire lifetime treating the sick and infirm. He even went as far to shave his head bald to better bond with those sick individuals being treated with radiation and chemotherapy. In his book, "Peace, Love and Healing" Bernie Siegel shows how our attitudes can dramatically influence our health and well being. He makes several humorous but true lists about how our attitudes make us sick or well.

How to Get Sick

1. Don't pay attention to your body. Eat plenty of junk food, drink too much, take too much drugs, have lots of unsafe sex with lots of different partners and above all, feel guilty about it. If you are over-stressed and over-tired, ignore it and keep pushing yourself.

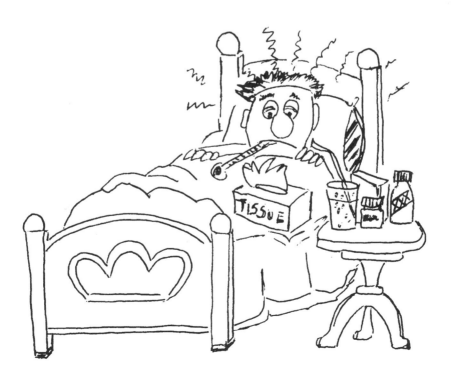

2. Cultivate the experience of your life as meaningless and of little value.

3. Do the things you don't like and avoid doing what you really want. Follow everyone else's opinion and advice, while seeing yourself as miserable and "stuck."

4. Be resentful and hyper-critical, especially towards yourself.

5. Fill your mind with dreadful pictures, and then obsess over them. Worry most of the time, if not all, of the time.

6. Avoid deep, lasting, intimate relationships.

7. Blame others for all of your problems.

8. Do not express your feelings and views openly and honestly. Other people wouldn't appreciate it. If at all possible, do not even know what your feelings are.

9. Shun anything that resembles a sense of humour. Life is no laughing matter.

10. Avoid making any changes which would bring you greater satisfaction and joy.

How to Get Sicker (If you are already sick)

1. Think about all the awful things that could happen to you. Dwell upon negative, fearful images.

2. Be depressed, self-pitying, envious and angry. Blame everyone and everything for your illness.

3. Read articles, books and newspapers, watch TV programs and listen to people who reinforce the viewpoint that there is NO HOPE. You are powerless to influence your fate.

4. Cut yourself off from other people. Regard yourself as a pariah. Lock yourself up in your room and contemplate death.

5. Hate yourself for having destroyed your life. Blame yourself mercilessly and incessantly.

6. Go see lots of different doctors. Run from on to another, spend half your time in waiting rooms, get lots of conflicting opinions and lots of experimental drugs and start one program after another without sticking to any.

7. Quit your job, stop work on any projects, give up all activities that bring you a sense of purpose and fun. See your life as essentially pointless and at an end.

8. Complain about your symptoms and if you associate with anyone, do so exclusively with other people who are unhappy and embittered. Reinforce each other's feelings of hopelessness.

9. Don't take care of yourself. What's the use? Try to get other people to do it for you and then resent them for doing a poor job.

10. Think how awful life is and how you might as well be dead. But make sure you are absolutely terrified of death, just to increase the pain.

The purpose of these "How to Get Sick" lists is to make you aware of certain negative attitudes and bad habits that impact your health. If you exhibit these attitudes or practice these habits then you will be promoting disease and ill health. You can take steps towards changing your attitudes and habits and improving your health and well being.

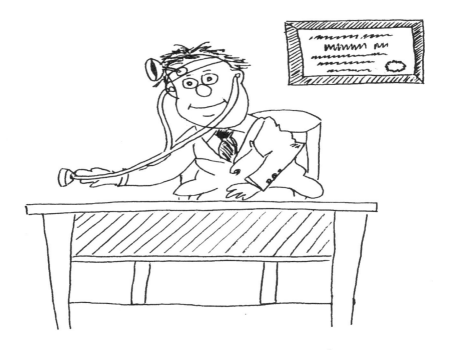

How to Stay Healthy (or get better)

1. Do things that bring you a sense of fulfillment, joy and purpose; that validate your worth. See your life as your own creation and strive to make it a positive one.

2. Pay close and loving attention to yourself, turning in to your needs on all levels. Take care of yourself, nourishing, supporting and encouraging others and yourself.

3. Release all negative emotions--resentment, envy, fear, sadness anger. Express your feeling appropriately, don't hold on to them. Forgive yourself.

4. Hold positive images and goals in your mind, pictures of what you truly want in your life. When fearful images arise, re-focus on images that evoke feelings of peace and joy.

5. Love yourself and love everyone else. Make loving the purpose and primary expression in your life.

6. Create fun, loving, honest relationships, allowing for the expression and fulfillment of needs for intimacy and security. Try to heal any wounds in past relationships, as with old lovers and your mother and father.

7. Make a positive contribution to your community, through some form of work or service that you value and enjoy.

8. Make a commitment to health and well-being and develop a belief in the possibility to total health. Develop your own healing program, drawing on the support and advice of experts without becoming enslaved to them.

9. Accept yourself and everything in your life as an opportunity for growth and learning. Be grateful. When you f--k up, forgive yourself, learn what you can and then move on.

10. Keep a sense of humour. Laugh at yourself and laugh with others. Laughter is a strong medicine

Please, if you want to become even healthier, pay particular attention to the last ten items.

Belief

Belief is acceptance of something we regard as true or good. A belief may be accepted with the scientific proof or on only faith alone. Faith is confidence or trust in our beliefs, without proof, such as religious belief. Examples of our belief system include our belief about God, this Universe, our purpose in life, morality, family, laws and rules and our behavior. Beliefs form the very core of our being. They influence every movement and behavior in our life. We may be hindered and hampered by negative beliefs that thwart our personal growth and prevent us from achieving our full potential. We may be empowered and encouraged by positive beliefs that stimulate our personal growth and propel us to achieve our goals. It is important to identify and examine our beliefs.

What do you believe and what are your beliefs?

1. I am my best me!
2. What you think about, you bring about
3. _____
4. Have a positive Mindset
5. The best revenge, is living well
6. The past is the past, leave it allown
7. Take control of your life
8. _____
9. _____
10. _____

David Suzuki and Chief Seattle

David Suzuki was a professor of genetics at the University of British Columbia while I was attending undergraduate school . He is the host and commentator of the awarding winning CBC show, The Nature of Things. He has also wrote several thought provoking books about man's influence on nature and the fragile ecological status of the world. From the book "Inventing the Future" there is the original translated testimony of Chief Seattle given to the assembly of tribes in 1854, as they prepared to sign a treaty with the white man. The shear eloquence of this speech is poetic. Read this classic oration and you will be impressed at the values, attitudes and beliefs of the Indian culture. We can learn from their wisdom and apply some of their knowledge in today's modern, secular life.

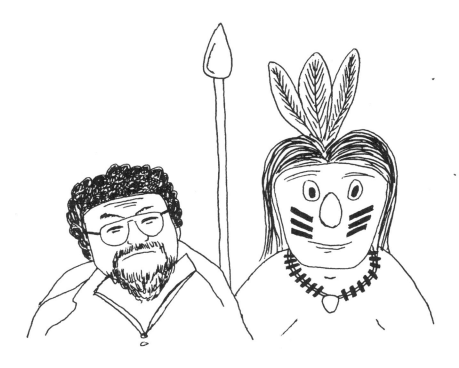

"How can you buy or sell the sky, the warmth of the land? The idea is strange to us. We do not own the freshness of the air and the sparkle of the water. Every part of this earth is sacred to my people. Every shining pine needle, every sandy shore, every mist in the dark woods, every clearing and humming insect is holy in the memory and experience of my people. The sap which courses through the trees carries the memories of the red man."

"The white man's dead forget the country of their birth when they go to walk among the stars. Our dead never forget this beautiful earth and it is part of us. The perfumed flowers are our sisters; the deer, the horse, the great eagle, these are our brothers.

The rocky crests, the juices of the meadows, the body heat of the pony, and man -- all belong to the same family."

"The ashes of our fathers are sacred. Their graves are holy ground, and so these hills, these trees, this portion of earth is consecrated to us. We known that the white man does not understand our ways. One portion of land is the same to him as the next, for he is a stranger who comes in the night and takes from the land whatever he needs. The earth is not his brother, but his enemy, and when he has conquered it, he moves on. He leaves his fathers' graves behind, and he does not care. He kidnaps the earth from his children. He does not care. His fathers' grave and his children's birthright are forgotten. He treats his mother, the earth, and his brother, the sky as things to be bought, plundered, sold like sheep or bright beads. His appetite will devour the earth and leave only a desert."

"I am a savage and I do not understand any other way. I have seen a thousand rotting buffaloes on the prairie, left by the white man who shot them from a passing train. I am a savage and I do not understand how the smoking iron horse can be more important than the buffalo that we kill only to stay alive."

"What is man without the beasts? If all the beasts were gone, men would die from great loneliness of spirit. For whatever happens to the beasts, soon happens to men. All things are interconnected."

"You must teach your children that the ground beneath their feet is the ashes of our grandfathers. So that they will respect the land, tell your children that the earth is rich with the lives of our kin. Teach your children what we have taught our children, the earth is our mother. Whatever befalls the earth befalls the sons of the earth. If men spit upon the ground, they spit upon themselves."

"Where is the thicket? Gone. Where is the eagle? Gone. And what is to say goodbye to the swift pony and the hunt? The

end of the living and the beginning of survival."

"This we know. The earth does not belong to man; man belongs to the earth. This we know. All things are connected like to blood which unites one family. All things are connected."

"Whatever befalls the earth befalls the sons of the earth. Man did not weave the web of life, he is merely a strand in it. Whatever he does to the web, he does to himself."

"The whites too shall pass; perhaps sooner that all other tribes. Continue to contaminate your bed, and you will one night suffocate in your own waste."

"When the last red man has vanished from the earth, and his memory is only the shadow of a cloud moving across the prairie, these shores and forests will still hold the spirits of my people. For they love this earth as the newborn loves its mother's heartbeat. So if we sell you our land, love it as we've loved it. Care for it as we've cared for it. Hold in your mind the memory of the land as it is when you take it. And with all your strength, with all your mind, with all your heart, preserve it for your children and love it."

Summary

1. Re-evaluate the beliefs you learned as a young child.
2. Clarify your physical and spiritual values.
3. Realize how your attitudes affect you.
4. Be aware of what attitudes make you sick and sicker.
5. Be aware of what attitudes make you well and healthy.
6. Clarify your beliefs.

Chapter 2

What Do You Want?

Imagine you are in a foreign country and you can't understand or read the language. You decide that you want to make a trip but you are not sure where you want to go. You get in your car and start driving down a road that you've never been on. You drive for the whole day, never arrive at your destination and finally decide your lost. Life is a lot like the challenge of driving in a foreign country. You must be clear on your destination and must have a plan to reach your goal. You must take action and persist until you reach your desired destination. You must be clear on what it is you want and then decide on a plan to achieve your goals.

What Are Your Desires?

In his book "The Seven Laws of Spiritual Success" Deepak Chopra uses his Indian heritage to explore at what is at the very core of human behavior. Sometimes in our fast-paced, secular lifestyle with many daily distractions and trivialities we lose sight of our inner desires. Your deepest, inner desires fuels your behavior and compels us to action. Rediscovering what it important to you at your personal core is important in determining what you want.

"You are what your deep, driving desire is.
As your desire is, so is your will.
As your will is, so is your deed.
As your deed is, so is your destiny."

How Far Have You Come?

Before you get caught up in achieving our goals it is important to make a personal assessment how far you've already come. Use the following outline to make an accurate assessment of how you've done in ten important areas of personal development from five years ago. Rate your progress on a scale of 0 to 10, with 0 being no progress, no achievement and no development and 10 being outstanding progress, achievement and development. The second part of this exercise is to write a little statement after your category and score outlining what you were like in each of these areas.

Category	Score	Statement
Physically		_____
		_____
Mentally		_____
		_____
Emotionally		_____
		_____
Appearance		_____
		_____
Relationships		_____
		_____
Living Environment		_____

_____

Socially   _____

_____

Spiritually   _____

_____

Career   _____

_____

Financially   _____

_____

Take inventory and see how you've done in the last five years. Identify your strengths and weaknesses. What are areas you've excelled in and what areas do you need improvement? For contrast repeat the same list while concentrating on your score only. How are you doing now in relationship from where you've come from? What areas have you excelled in and what areas do you need to concentrate on?

Goals

Before you decide where you want to go, you must decide on what you want? Personal goals are a way of defining what you want. A goal is simply a marking post that defines the end of the race or an aim or a purpose. It defines what you want to achieve, what you want to accomplish and where you want to go. Goals are useful in identifying your outcome and gauging your growth and development. Sometimes our whole behavior is the result of our defining goals. Our actions and our course in life may be a result of our desire to achieve our goals. Before we identify our goals it is important to understand why we have goals. Goals are useful landmarks in gauging our growth and development. Goals can be loosely defined as to which part of the human psyche they develop. Goals can be physical, mental, emotional and spiritual. Physical goals can be career or work oriented, materialistic or health oriented. All goals are important and it is important to define all goals.

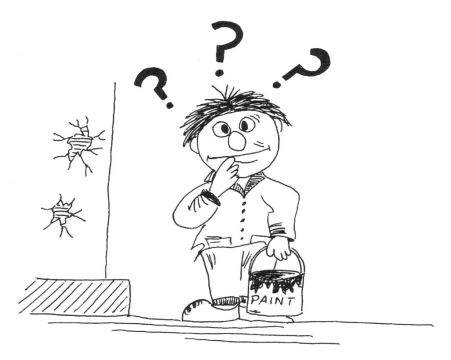

Personal Development Goals

One the following list identify ten of your most important personal development goals. Personal development goals include things you would like to learn, subjects you would like to study, skills you want to master, traits you would like to develop, things you would like to do. After you list each personal development goal, put a time line on achieving this goal. Remember goals are dreams with a deadline. Identify your most important personal goal that you want to achieve within one year. Circle this goal. Review your list.

1. _____

2. _____

3. _____

4. _____

5. _____

6. _____

7. _____

8. _____

9. _____

10. _____

Career or Financial Goals

One the following list identify ten of your most important career or financial goals. Career or financial goals include what job or career you would like to embark on, how much money you would like to earn this year, what company you would like to work for, what your net worth is, money management goals and investments you would like to make. After you list each career or financial goal, put a time line on achieving that goal. Identify your most important career or financial goal that you want to achieve within one year. Circle this goal. Review your list.

1. _____

2. _____

3. _____

4. _____

5. _____

6. _____

7. _____

8. _____

9. _____

10. _____

Health and Fitness Goals

On the following list identify ten of your most important personal health and fitness goals. Health and fitness goals include what physical activities you want to embark on, what spiritual or emotional activities that improve your health, what illness you want to avoid, what disease you want to overcome. After you list each health and fitness goal, put a time limit on achieving that goal. Identify your most important health and fitness goal that you want to achieve within one year. Circle this goal. Review your list.

1. _____

2. _____

3. _____

4. _____

5. _____

6. _____

7. _____

8. _____

9. _____

10. _____

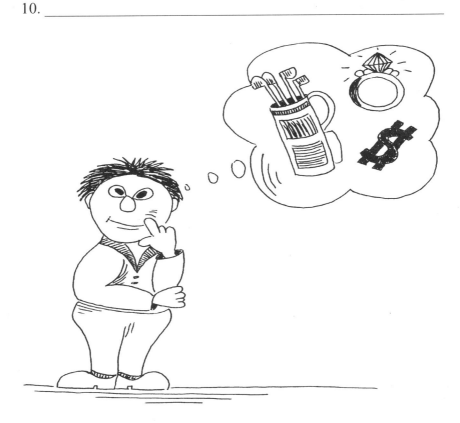

Recreation or Play Goals

On the following list identify ten of your most important recreation or play goals. Pay no attention to monetary restrictions. Identify ten toys, play things or adventures you would like to have or embark on. Recreation or play goals include anything you would like to build, create or purchase, things you would like to attend or places you want to go. After you list each goal put a time limit on achieving that goal. Identify your most important toy or play goal that you want to achieve within one year. Circle that goal. Review your list.

1. _____

2. _____

3. _____

4. _____

5. _____

6. _____

7. _____

8. _____

9. _____

10. _____

Contribution Goals

One the following list identify ten of your most important contribution goals. Contribution goals are among the most inspiring and compelling of all goals. Contribution goals include what legacy you would like to leave behind, what contribution you want to make to society or the world, what difference you want to make in the world or what you want to remembered the most for. After you list each goal put a time limit on achieving that goal. Identify your most important contribution goal that you would like to achieve within one year. Circle that goal. Review your list.

1. _____

2. _____

3. _____

4. _____

5. _____

6. _____

7. _____

8. _____

9. _____

10. _____

Purpose of Goal Setting

The whole purpose of goals is to gauge and measure your growth and development. It is important to realize that achieving our goals are not the most important things in life. The means of achieving our goals are more important than the goals themselves. The pathway we choose, the struggle that ensues, the hardships we endure, the lessons learned, the skills we acquire, and the person we become are defining points of human behavior. Our goals allows us to grow, develop and change. Achieving our goals allows us the measure and assess our growth and development. The type of person we become while following a pathway to achieve our goals is more defining that achieving a goal itself. It is important to reflect and reaffirm the purpose of our goals. The whole purpose of our goals should be reflected by our personal mission statement. Our goals should be a statement of the type of person we want to become. We should strive to be that person while trying to achieve our goals.

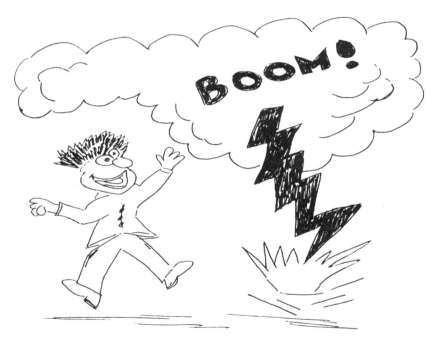

Benefits of Goals

The ultimate benefit of achieving our goals is to not to ourselves but rather to mankind, the world, mother nature and the universe. On a superficial level goals can selfish and self-absorbing. But the underlying purpose of our goals is to allow us to make contributions and gifts back to the universe which is responsible for giving us life and our existence. Don't lose sight of this important statement. In our secular, materialistic society we often lose sight of the importance and ultimate purpose of our goals. Making a lot of money, becoming wealthy or a millionaire, retiring early, and gaining material possessions are not the ultimate purpose of our goals. Making a lot of money for yourself or gaining a lot of material wealth for yourself is not the ultimate purpose of our goals. Using your money, wealth and possessions for the benefit of others, the world and the universe is by far a greater and satisfying purpose. It is important to reaffirm the purpose of our goals and how achieving our goals will benefit others and the universe.

Personal Mission Statement

A personal mission statement is a short statement that identifies what type of person you want to become and develop into. It summarizes your most important values, it influences your attitude and beliefs and is reflected in our goals and what things you want to achieve. Write a short personal mission statement that identifies what your mission or purpose is in life.

_____

_____

_____

_____

_____

_____

Pathway to Success

In his best-selling book, "Unlimited Power" Anthony Robbins outlines the consistent pathway to achieving your goals. The formula is virtually the same for all goals. Follow the steps as outlined. Take action. And you will be on your way to achieve what it is you want.

1. Define precisely what it is you want. Be specific as possible. Define your goals in realistic terms.

2. Set time limits to your goals. Otherwise your goals will be just dreams. You must set a realistic time period in which to achieve your goals. Be somewhat lenient, but also be firm in your dates.

3. Outline a variety of different pathways that you can use to achieve your goals. Be creative, but also realistic and practical. Brainstorm on different pathways that you can possibly use. It helps to write these pathways down while you think about them.

4. Take the action necessary to achieve your goals. Action must be taken in a specific time period. Otherwise your goals will be just dreams without time periods. Nobody can force you to take the action necessary to achieve your goals. Most people know what to do, some people know how to do it and even less people take action and apply themselves.

5. Be flexible to change if the results you achieve aren't consistent with your goals. Adaptability is an important skill that is necessary to achieve your goals. It makes no sense to take consistent action, if the action does not allow you to meet your goals. You must be willing to change your actions if necessary.

6. Know your results are consistent with your life's purpose and are reflected in your personal mission statement. Goals are not the end to the means. It is the means; the pathways and struggles, that allow us further growth and development that are important.

Summary

1. Take inventory of how far you have come?
2. What are your personal development goals?
3. What are your career or financial goals?
4. What are your health or fitness goals?
5. What are your toy or play goals?
6. What are your contribution goals?
7. Write a personal mission statement.
8. Follow the pathway to success.

Chapter 3

Making Things Happen

You may have good intentions. You may have outstanding attitudes, values and beliefs. You may have tremendous goals. If you don't apply yourself; if you don't make things happen, then you will not achieve your goals. Most people fail to achieve their goals in life because of lack of action, procrastination and inconsistent effort. To achieve your goals, you must first have goals, write them down, put a time line on them and then take logical and practical steps to achieving them. There is no short cut to success. You must have consistent effort, apply yourself, work hard and deal with the pressures and frustrations of trying to achieve your goals.

Start With Yourself

In an effort to make things happen, you must start with yourself. You are responsible for your ability to take action and to achieve your goals. You are largely accountable for your successes and failures. There is nobody to blame for your lack of effort but yourself.

From the book "Chicken Soup for the Soul" by Jack Canfield and Mark Victor Hansen comes the following quotation. This statement was written on the tomb of an Anglican Bishop in the crypts of Westminister Abbey:

"When I was young and free and my imagination had no limits, I dreamed of changing the world. As I grew older and wiser, I discovered the world would not change, so I shortened my sights somewhat and decided to change my country. But it, too seem immovable."

"As I grew my twilight years, in one last desperate attempt, I settled for changing only my family, those closest to me, but alas, they would have none of it. "

"And now as I lie on my deathbed, I suddenly realized: If I had only changed myself first, then by example I would have changed my family. From their inspiration and encouragement, I would have then been able to better my country and, who knows, I may have even changed the world."

An Example of Persistence

One of the most important factors in making things happen is the ability to consistently produce effort and persist in the face of adversity. Probably one of the greatest example of persistence is Abraham Lincoln. If you want to learn about somebody who didn't quit, look no further. When you become frustrated and discouraged think about Abraham Lincoln and the adversity he faced to become one of the great American presidents.

"Born into poverty, Lincoln was faced with defeat throughout his life. He lost eight elections, twice failed in business and suffered a nervous breakdown. He could have quit many times -- but he didn't and because he didn't quit, he became one of the greatest presidents in the history of the United States. Lincoln was a champion and never gave up. Here is a sketch of Lincoln's road to the White House."

"In 1816, his family was forced out of their home. He had to work to support them. In 1818, his mother died. In 1831, he

failed at business. In 1832, he ran for state legislature and lost. In 1832, he also lost his job and wanted to go law school but couldn't afford it. In 1833, he borrowed some money from a friend to begin a business and by the end of the year he was bankrupt. He spent the next 17 years of his life paying off this debt. In 1834, he ran for state legislature and won this time. In 1835, he was engaged to be married, but his sweetheart died and his heart was broken. In 1836, he had a total nervous breakdown and was in bed for six months. In 1838, he sought to become speaker of the state legislature and was defeated. In 1840, he sought to become elector and was defeated. In 1843, he ran for congress and lost. In 1846, he ran for congress again and won this time. He went to Washington, D.C. and did a good job. In 1848, he ran for re-election in congress and was defeated. In 1849, he sought the job of land officer in his home state and was rejected. In 1854, he ran for senate of the United States and lost. In 1856, he sought vice-presidential nomination at his party's national convention and got less than 100 votes. In 1858, he ran for the U.S. senate again and lost again. In 1860, he was elected president of the United States."

After losing a senate race, Abraham Lincoln was quoted as saying "the path was worn and slippery. My foot slipped from under me, knocking the other out of the way, but I recovered and said to myself, It's a slip and not a fall."

Can You Handle The Critics?

A critic is a person who offers an opinion or evaluation, good or bad, about our behavior and action. While positive criticism can be beneficial and encouraging negative criticism can be discouraging and stifling. You must learn to deal with negative criticism and not let it affect your behavior or prevent you from achieving your goals. Another American president, Theodore Roosevelt offered this advice about being able to handle the critics, trying your best and sticking to your goals.

"It is not the critic who counts, not the man who points out how the strong man stumbles or where the doer of deeds could have done them better. The credit belongs to the man who is actually in the arena, whose face is marred by dust and sweat and blood, who strives valiantly, who errs and comes short again and again, because there is no effort without error and shortcomings, who knows the great devotion, who spends himself in a worthy cause, who at best knows in the end the high achievement of triumph and who at worse, if he fails while daring greatly, knows his place shall never be with those timid and cold souls who know neither victory or defeat."

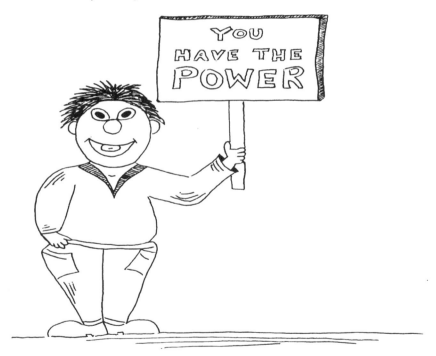

Try Something Different

Eventhough you may work hard and are persistent and you handle the critics, it is sometimes necessary to try something different in your approach to getting what you want. Many people get locked into a rut of trying harder without trying smarter. Trying harder does not always work. Sometimes we need to do something radically different to achieve greater levels of success. We need to break out of our paradigm prisons, our habit patterns and our comfort zones. Take time to re-evaluate exactly what it is you want and your approach to achieving it. As the old saying goes, instead of beating your head against the wall, it is sometimes easier to just walk around it.

Seven Habits of Success

One of the most important factors of getting what you want is to develop habits that are consistent with success. Anthony Robbins is the brash, motivational guru on late night television who wrote the bestselling book "Unlimited Power." I strongly encourage you to read this book. It is one of the best personal self-improvement books I have ever read. This is a summary of the seven habits of success from his book. Read them over, ponder them and try to consistently apply them in every day life.

1. Everything happens for a reason or purpose.
2. No such thing as failure.
3. Take responsibility.
4. It is not necessary to know everything.
5. People are your greatest asset.
6. Work is play.
7. There is no success without commitment.

Five Skills For Achieving Your Goals

Anthony Robbins goes on to further elaborate five skills for achieving your goals. As you attempt to make things happen you will undoubtedly encounter trials and frustrations along your way. You must develop skills to handle frustration, rejection, pressure and complacency.

1. Learn how to handle frustration.
2. Learn how to handle rejection.
3. Learn how to handle pressure.
4. Learn how to handle complacency.
5. Always give more than you expect to receive.

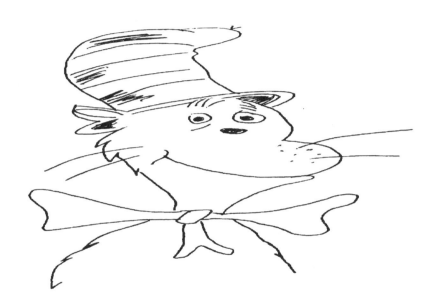

Success and Dr. Suess

I remember as a young child reading the now classic book by Dr. Suess called "Green Eggs and Ham." There is much wisdom found in children stories that can be applied to adult life. The following poem by Dr. Suess is quoted from a senior student's valedictorian speech about meeting the challenges of the future and achieving your goals.

"You have brains in your head.
You have feet on your shoes
You can steer yourself .
Any direction you chose
...So be sure when you step.

Step with care and great tact
And remember that life's
a great balancing act...
And you will succeed?
Yes, you will indeed
98 and 3/4 per cent guaranteed."

Think You Can

The following poem is from the inspirational book "Chicken Soup For the Soul" by Jack Canfield and Mark Victor Hansen. One of the most important factors in achieving success is to use your state of mind. You must believe in yourself and think that you can achieve your goals and you are successful.

"If you think you are beaten, you are.
If you think you dare not, you don't.
If you like to win, but you think you can't,
It is almost certain you won't."

"If you think you'll lose, you're lost.
for out in the world we find,
Success begins with a fellow's will--
It's all a state of mind."

"If you think you are outclassed, you are,
You've got to think high to rise,
You've got to be sure of yourself before,
You can ever win a prize."

"Life's battles don't always go,
To the stronger or faster man,
But soon or late the man who wins,
Is the one WHO THINKS HE CAN."

Call Of The Wild

One of my earlier childhood heroes was Jack London, the intrepid author and adventurer, who wrote such classics as "Call of the Wild" and "White Fang." He spent some time in the Alaskan frontier in the early 20th century. He encountered many of the hardships and tribulations associated with that environment. While in college I kept one of his inspirational quotations on my bulletin board and read it frequently. It exemplifies the attitude of hard work and consistent effort.

"Don't loaf and invite inspiration; light out after it with a club and if you don't get it, you nontheless get something that looks remarkably like it. Work all the time. Find out about this earth, this universe, this force and matter from the maggot to the godhead. And by this I mean work for your philosophy of life. It doesn't hurt how wrong your philosophy is, so long as you have one and have it well."

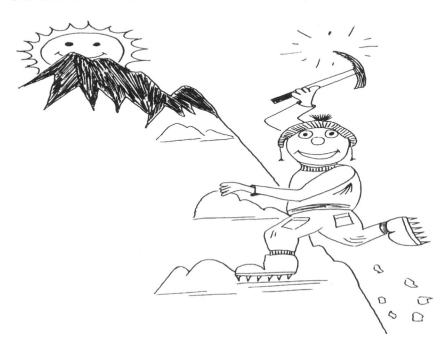

Take Action

One of the most important factors in making things happen is the ability to take action. You must take consistent action in the quest of achieving your goals and becoming successful. Goals without action will always remain dreams. Don't procrastinate. be persistent, take action and make things happen.

Summary

To make things happen you must:

1. Start with yourself.
2. Be persistent.
3. Handle the critics.
4. Try something different, if necessary.
5. Develop the habits of success.
6. Practice the skills of achieving your goals.
7. Believe in yourself.
8. Think that you can achieve your goals.
9. Work hard and take action.

Chapter 4

Time Management and Problem Solving

You need certain basic skills in work and life to be successful. Time management and problem solving are necessary skills. Developing, cultivating and nurturing these skills takes time and practice. They are essential for getting what you want in life. They are useful skills in achieving optimal health and well being.

Seven Basic Skills

Seven basic skills of time management are outlined in the book "Managing Your Mind" by Gillian Butler and Tony Hope. They show you how to develop and cultivate these skills. These fundamental skills enable you to improve your mood, the way you feel about yourself, your work and productivity. As with any skill the more you practice the better you will become. You will manage your time better and be able to solve problems easier.

1. Manage yourself and your time.
2. Face the problem.
3. Treat yourself right.
4. Solve the problem.
5. Keep things in perspective.
6. Build your self-confidence and esteem.
7. Learn to relax.

Effective time management begins with managing yourself. You must treat yourself right and take steps towards building self-confidence and self-esteem. You must learn to relax and avoid getting stressed out about your problems. You must take steps towards effective problem solving. Begin by identifying the problem and then take steps towards solving the problem. Try to cultivate these skills of effective time management on a daily basis.

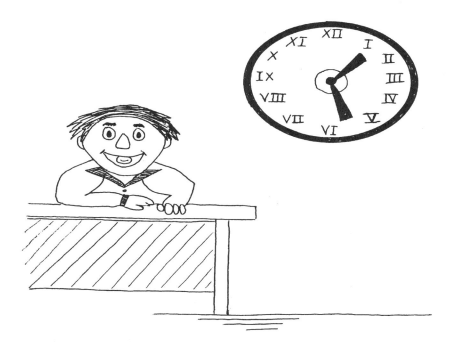

Time Management

We all have only 24 hours in each day. How you manage your time for all your daily activities depends on effective time management. One of the most important principles of time management is that you spend your time doing those things you value the most or that help you achieve your goals. It is therefore important to know what your values, beliefs and goals are. You can clarify your values, beliefs and goals by imagining what a close friend relative or colleague would say about you.

What type of person would you be described as by a close friend, relative or colleague?

_____

_____

_____

_____

_____

What Is Important To You?

The central principle of time management is spend your time doing the things you value or help you achieve your goals. It is obviously important to know your goals and values. Reaffirm your goals and values by reviewing them daily. Ask yourself the question, "what is really important to you right now?"

What is important to you, right now? What problems do you want to solve?

_____

_____

_____

_____

_____

_____

Tools For Time Management

Tools are a practical implement you can use to improve your time management. Like skills, they must be developed and practiced to be effective.

- Stop procrastinating.
- Develop and follow a routine.
- Learn to say "no."
- Put things in perspective.
- Cut things up into small pieces.
- Avoid the curse of perfectionism.
- Start and end appointments.
- Make time to plan.

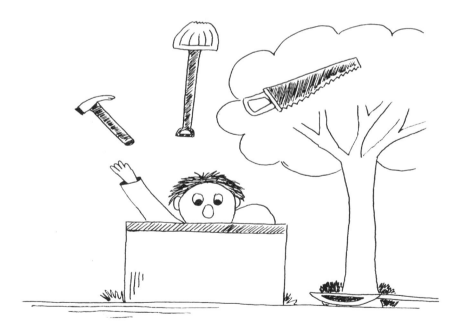

Procrastination means to delay, avoid or put off doing an activity. To stop procrastinating means to directly face your problem and make a whole hearted effort to solve it. To avoid committing yourself to too many projects or appointments you must learn to say no and mean it. Take steps to identify what is important to you and say "no" to things that are not important to you. Put things in perspective by asking yourself the following questions: What needs to be done right now? What is important to me right now?

To avoid being overwhelmed by a large, foreboding problem, break the problem into small chunks. Take small steps to solve this problem. After you have taken several small steps, the sum of the steps will add up and you will be well on your way towards solving the big problem. Avoid the curse of perfectionism. Avoid getting in the trap of trying to make the perfect masterpiece of one problem or project. Do your best for a specific period of time, then move on. Do not get stuck in the rut of trying to be perfect. Keep a timetable by starting and ending all appointments. Once the appointment has ended do not dwell on it, move on and apply your energy to other problems or other areas of your life. Make a time plan, write down your goals and set a time line for achieving your goals.

Avoidance

Avoiding problems or issues is like sweeping dust under a rug. It helps to avoid the immediate problem, at least for a moment or two, but sooner or later the problem will come back and haunt you. Facing our problems or issues is rarely as alarming as we make them out to be in our mind and imagination. Avoidance of problems and issues is unproductive and interferes with effective time management. It can make the problem worse. It can create new problems and can interfere with other aspects of our life. Facing difficulties can be hard. The first step is to recognize that there is a problem or issue. The second step is to identify the problem or issue. Only then can you take steps to work out or remedy the problem. It will help you decide what to do next. Catching the problem early enough helps you to find an effective solution earlier. They will have less chance of growing into imaginary monsters and mountains. Most problems shrink in size and intensity when we look at them directly. Recognize that there is a problem, identify the problem and decide upon effective ways of solving the problem or issue.

Write down five problems that you have been avoiding or procrastinating about for a long time. Circle the problem you would like to solve right now.

_____

_____

_____

_____

_____

_____

Problem Solving

There are specific fundamental steps that can be taken to solve any problem regardless of what it is. In their book "Managing Your Mind", Gillian Butler and Tony Hope outline the simple steps of problem solving.

- Identify the problem clearly.
- Generate as many solutions to the problem as possible. It does not matter what the solution is or how preposterous it sounds. Do not reject any solution that comes to you.
- Take steps toward solving the problem.
- Select a solution to your problem from your list.
- Try it out.
- Evaluate what happens. Does it solve the problem effectively?
- If the solution does solve the problem, you are successful.

- If the solution does not solve the problem, try a different solution.
- Persist until you feel better.

The Problem:

_____

_____

_____

_____

Possible Solutions:

_____

_____

_____

_____

_____

_____

_____

Select A Solution:

_____

Try it out.

Evaluate what happens.

If the solution is not successful, then try a different solution.

Persist until you feel better and have the results you desire.

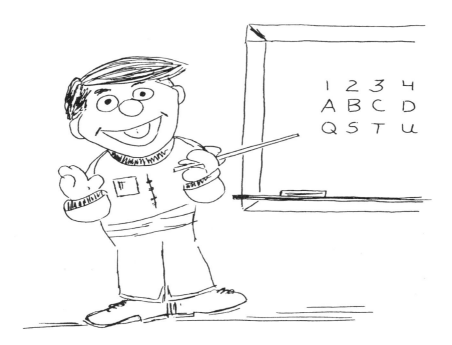

Important But Not Urgent

One of the most useful things I learned from the book "The 7 Habits of Highly Effective People" by Stephen Covey is to categorize your problems or tasks as to their importance and urgency. Most people tend to be crisis oriented. They focus their time and attention to problems or tasks that bear urgent action. While urgent problems or tasks may by important or not that important. As an example, if your car breaks down and prevents you from going to work, the problem is important and urgent and requires your immediate attention and energy. However, if your phone bill is due, the problem is important but not that urgent. All problems can be classified as to their importance and urgency. While it is vital to deal with problems that are important and urgent, it is also useful and productive to deal with problems that are important but not urgent.

Write down three problems that are important and require your immediate attention.

_____

_____

_____

_____

_____

Write down five problems that are important but not that urgent.

_____

_____

_____

_____

_____

_____

_____

_____

Effective problem solving and time management is necessary for attending to all problems including those that are important but not that urgent. While we tend to focus most of our attention and time on problems that are important and urgent, it is also important to focus on problems that our important but not urgent. By focusing some time and energy on problems that are important but not urgent you will greatly improve your productivity in daily life.

Summary

1. Practice the seven basic skills for time management and problem solving.
2. Evaluate what is important to you and what problems you want to solve.
3. Use the tools of effective time management.
4. Avoid procrastination and denial.
5. Take steps towards effective problem solving.
6. Try a solution out.
7. Evaluate what happens.
8. Persist until you get the results you desire.
9. Identify problems according their importance and urgency.

Chapter 5

Managing Your Emotions

We, as humans are emotional creatures. Emotions are particular ways of feeling or being excited such as love, hate, joy, awe, fear, grief and happiness. Feelings are particular sensations that you experience. Human behavior including our attitudes, beliefs and goals is often influenced by our emotional state. Emotions can be positive and negative. While positive emotions are uplifting and nourishing, negative emotions are depleting and discouraging. When we experience negative emotions, they tend to affect human behavior much more adversely than positive emotions. Negative emotions tend to influence are actions more strongly than positive emotions. It is important to identify and realize how emotions affect how you feel and affect your behavior.

Write down emotions, positive or negative, that you experience on a daily basis.

1. _____

2. _____

3. _____

4. _____

5. _____

6. _____

7. _____

8. _____

9. _____

10. _____

The Giant Within

Anthony Robbins is the brash, motivational guru on late night television. In his book "Awaken the Giant Within" he outlines strategies for mastering your emotions, taking charge of your life and fulfilling your full potential. He points out the ten negative emotions that adversely affect our behavior and presents the ten positive emotions that are nurturing and healing. He defines the emotion, shows how it affects us and outlines effective strategies for overcoming the it's ill effects. He also shows the benefits of positive emotions on our health and well being.

Ten Negative Emotions

1. Anger
2. Fear
3. Discomfort
4. Hurt
5. Frustration
6. Disappointment
7. Guilt
8. Inadequacy
9. Overwhelm
10. Loneliness

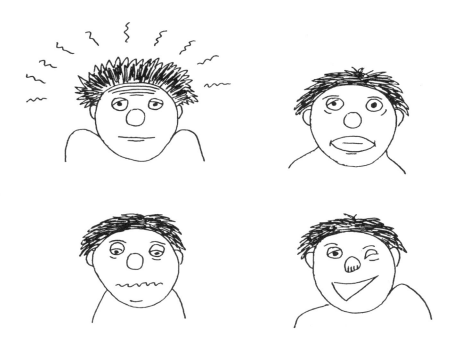

Anger

Anger is a strong emotion aroused by a sense of of injury or wrong.

The emotion anger is evoked when we feel angry about someone or something who has violated our inner core values and beliefs. Anger leads to provocation and resentment. Anger can lead to other regretful emotional responses such as verbal yelling or physical action. We are typically angered by those individuals that we love and are close to us.

To overcome anger you must define what it is we are angry about. Ask yourself the following questions. Who or what has violated are inner core being? Is anger the appropriate response for this situation? Are we over-reacting to the situation in an inappropriate manner? Realize that you may have misinterpreted the situation. Eventhough you feel someone has violated you, your rules or standards do not govern all behavior in the universe. In the big picture does this violation actually matter? Will it matter one hour from now, a day from now or even next year? What can I learn from this?

Communicate your sense of violation to the other person or parties involved. Don't do this by yelling or screaming. This may be a highly inappropriate response for the situation. Do it rationally and calmly. Let the other person or parties know what and why it is you feel violated. Finally a change of attitude may be necessary to overcoming this emotion. Change your way of perceiving, change your response and change your behavior if necessary.

Fear

Fear is a strong emotion aroused by impending alarm or dread or about possible evil danger to you. Fear may evoke other emotions such as anxiety, awe, reverence or alarm.

The emotion fear is evoked when you anticipate that something may happen to you in the future. Fear is usually in response to impending change. The change may be good or bad. It may be evil, dangerous or harmful to you, but it can also be positive and beneficial. Fear is a reactionary emotion that something is about to happen. Some change is eminent and be prepared for it.

To overcome fear you must identify what it is that is making you fearful. Realize that fear is actually an emotional response to impending change. If it is a rationally based fear, then change your actions, so that you don't produce the fearful response. If it is an irrational, unfounded response then continue with your actions with the intent of producing the desired result. Change may be imminent, necessary and beneficial. If you need to take action then take it. Have faith that your actions will produce the results that are fruitful and beneficial. Remember there is nothing to fear, but fear itself.

Discomfort

Discomfort is a nagging emotion that signals that something is just not quite right. It is not a highly intense emotion like anger or fear but is real enough to create an uncomfortable feeling.

The emotion discomfort is evoked when you are bored, impatient, uneased, distressed or mildly embarrassed. You need to address this emotion. Perhaps something you are doing or feeling is not producing the results you want.

To overcome discomfort is to first identify what is producing this emotion. Redefine exactly what it is you want. Change your state of mind or your way of perceiving what is going on to you. Use your skills to try a different approach to solving your problems or achieving your goals.

Hurt

Hurt is a strong emotion characterized by a sense of loss or wrongdoing. Hurt is evoked when we feel somebody has or hasn't done something that has fallen short of our expectations.

The emotion hurt is evoked when your expectations are not met; goals were not achieved. You may also feel that somebody has wronged you by doing so.

To overcome hurt you must identify where your expectations have fallen short and subsequent loss has been generated. You can reaffirm hurtful emotion and look at the big picture. Is it really hurt and have you really lost something or have you misinterpreted their actions? Are you judging the outcome too soon? You can approach the person or parties involved and communicate your sense of loss. By communicating your hurtful emotion you are really addressing your sense of loss.

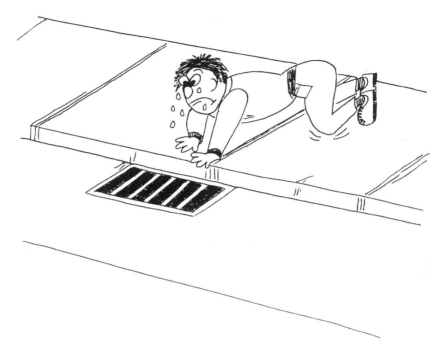

Frustration

Frustration is an emotion that signals that our actions are not producing the results we desire. Frustration compels us to move forward and change our actions.

The emotion is evoked when you feel that you are not achieving the desired results through your actions. You could be doing better than you currently are. And the results of your shortcomings produces frustration.

To overcome frustration you must identify exactly what it is that is frustrating you. Realize that frustration is a positive sign that is signaling that something is going to change so that you can be producing the desired results. Brainstorm or write down possible solutions to your problem. Change your way of acting or responding and try a different approach.

Disappointment

Disappointment is an emotion beyond frustration. It is characterized by an emotional let down. Your actions have failed to produce the results you desired.

The emotion disappointment is evoked when you are probably not going to achieve the results or goals you originally set.

To overcome disappointment you must re-evaluate exactly what your goals are. Try to identify why your actions have not produced the desired results. What can you learn from these actions or trials? If need be set a new goal or target. Realize that you may be too hard on yourself or you may be judging too soon. Realize the situation is not over yet . Cultivate patience and be persistent. Get the information or training you need to achieve your goals.

Guilt

Guilt is a strong emotion that makes us feel remorseful or shameful. Guilt is evoked when we realize that we have done something wrong or hurtful

The emotion guilt is evoked when you have violated one of your personal standards or ethics. Your actions have produced results that are contrary to your higher personal rules of conduct.

To overcome guilt you must identify what action has produced the guilty emotion. You have to redefine exactly why we feel guilty about this action. Sometimes you feel guilty about actions that you really shouldn't feel guilty about. If this is the case then change your emotional state, move on and forget about it. You really shouldn't feel guilty about it at all. On-the-other-hand maybe your actions have violated our own personal standards. Acknowledge that you have made a mistake. Learn from your previous actions. Forgive yourself and make sure your future actions don't produce the same results. Follow a different path that produces actions that don't violate your personal standards and ethics.

Inadequacy

Inadequacy is an emotion that you have fallen short of your expectations and you are not producing the results you could.

The emotion inadequacy is evoked when you don't have the necessary skills to achieve the results you or somebody else desires of you. You need more training, information, understanding or confidence.

To overcome inadequacy you must define why you feel inadequate? Is this the appropriate emotion for the situation at hand or are you over-reacting too quickly? What skills or technical information are you lacking? Do you need more love, understanding or encouragement? Ask for the support you need. Find a role model that shows you how or helps you develop your skills or provides you with the necessary encouragement. Get coaching and training if you need it. Change your approach, redefine your goals or change your actions altogether.

Overwhelm

Grief, depression and helplessness are merely expressions of feeling overloaded or overwhelmed. Grief happens when you feel like there is no empowering meaning for something that has happened or that your life is being negatively impacted by people, events or forces that are outside your control. People in this state become overwhelmed and often begin to feel that nothing can change the situation, that the problem is too big, it's permanent, pervasive and personal.

The emotion overwhelm is evoked when you are overloaded or

overwhelmed and you may be trying to deal with too many things at once. You need to re-evaluate what is most important to you in this situation.

To overcome overwhelm you must decide out of all the things you are currently dealing with in your life right now, what is the absolute, most important thing for you to focus on? Now write down all the things that are most important for you to accomplish and put them in order of priority. Just putting them down on paper will allow you to begin to feel a sense of control in what is going on around you. Tackle the first and most important thing on your list. Persist until you've accomplished or mastered what you've set out to do. When you feel that it is appropriate to let go of an overwhelming emotion like grief, start focusing on what you can control and realize that there must be some empowering, enlightening or enabling meaning to it all, even if you can't comprehend it at the moment. If you become overloaded or overwhelmed you must realize that you have the power to change what you are focusing on to help you deal with the situation at hand.

Loneliness

Loneliness is a feeling of being alone, apart, separate or dissociated from others. Everyone has felt this emotion from time to time in their lives.

The emotion loneliness is evoked when you feel lonely, disconnected and cut off from other people around you. The connections that you want to make and the communication you need are not happening.

To overcome loneliness you must realize that you can reach out and make a connection to someone someplace at any moment. There are wonderful, beautiful and caring people everywhere who want to make a connection. It is important to realize what type of connection that you need to make. Maybe you need some social friendship or a friend to share and talk to or maybe the type of connection you need to make is with your God or creator or maybe the connection you need to make is intimate and sexual. Remind yourself that being or feeling lonely is a wake up call that really means you really care about and love other things and people. Take immediate action, reach out and make that connection. Remember to have a friend is to be a friend.

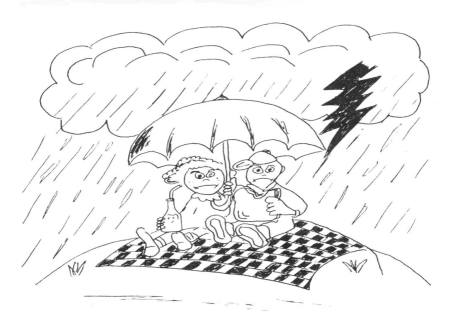

What Negative Emotions Affect You?

It is a fact of human psychology that negative emotions tend to govern our behavior more so than positive ones. We will go to great lengths to avoid negative feelings more so than positive feelings.

Write down one of the preceding negative emotions that you most strongly identify with. In your own words write down why you experience this emotion, how it affects you negatively and what solution you can generate to deal with it?

_____

_____

_____

_____

_____

Now write down the second most common negative emotion you experience, why it occurs, how it affects you and how you can deal with it.

_____

_____

_____

_____

_____

Ten Positive Emotions

1.   Love
2.   Thankfulness
3.   Curiosity
4.   Passion
5.   Determination
6.   Flexibility
7.   Confidence
8.   Joyfulness
9.   Vitality
10.   Contribution

Love

Love is the universal emotion of genuine warmth and caring that binds us all together. Love can literally melt away all negative emotions, instantaneously. We all crave for love. We seek it out and we want to express it and give it away. Love involves caring about other people, things in this world and a universal creator or Godhead. Love is the most positive, uplifting and unifying emotion in the universe. We must show love towards ourselves and others on a daily basis. By showing and expressing love you will feel good about yourself, others and the world we live in.

Thankfulness

Thankfulness is a special form of love that involves us expressing our personal heartfelt thanks for something. Thankfulness means saying thanks and truly meaning it. In our fast paced, secular lifestyle we often overlook the simple things in life. We often forget to be grateful for many things. We should be truly grateful for these simple things including food, shelter, clothing and even life itself. Showing thankfulness in the form of gratitude is an important aspect of daily existence.

Curiosity

Curiosity is emotion of wonder or awe. If you want to cultivate curiosity watch a child at play exploring his or her world. Children express true curiosity as they learn about the incredible world around them. Children want to learn why and how. They are truly amazed at the beauty and incredible diversity and complexity of the world. As we grow older into adulthood we lose our sense of curiosity. A sure cure for boredom is to cultivate curiosity and learn something new about this universe. Try to learn and enjoy the many unusual and interesting aspects of life in this universe.

Passion

Passion is an intense feeling or powerful emotion about something. You can be passionate about an emotion such as love and hate directed toward a person, an object, an idea or philosophy. A passionate person exudes enthusiasm about an object of interest or love in their life. When you are passionate about something you literally bubble over with exuberance. In our day-to-day lives at work and home we are often lacklustre about our affairs. We lack passion about our work and home life. When you really believe in something or somebody so strong, intense and powerful you begin to show passion. The real challenge in our lives is to show passion on a daily basis.

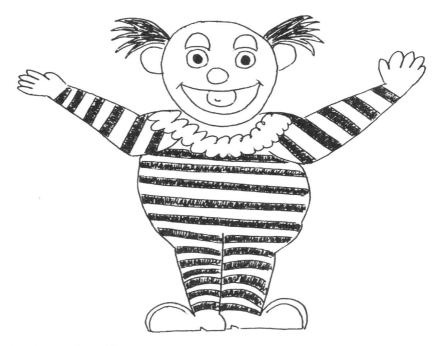

Determination

Determination is an unwavering commitment to achieve what you've set out to do. Determination is the ability to be consistent, working towards your goals. Determination is the ability to be unwavering in the face of adversity. Determination means sticking to your original plan or goals. Without determination you can never achieve your goals.

Flexibility

Flexibility is the ability to change and adapt to different circumstances as they present themselves. Flexibility means to bend and mold without breaking apart. You must be flexible to achieve your goals and be successful. You can have outstanding goals and have the utmost determination to achieve these goals, but without flexibility you may be prevented from achieving your goals. You may have to change your goals, your approach or your attitude if the situation warrants it. Sometimes being flexible is smarter than simply being determined and working harder.

Confidence

Confidence is the ability to believe in yourself and your abilities. Confidence involves trust and self-assurance with who you are and what you are doing. Confidence means that you not only have goals and are determined that you will achieve them, but also that you are confident you will achieve them. Be confident about yourself, who you are, what you believe and your abilities to achieve your goals and dreams.

Joyfulness

Joyfulness is a happy and cheerful attitude. While we are occasionally joyful about certain events and aspects about our life, we often lack true cheerfulness on a daily basis. Joyfulness, like happiness, is a state of mind. Since we can influence our emotions through what we think, I believe you can choose to be cheerful. Cultivate joyfulness today. Have a cheerful attitude and be happy and joyful about who you are and what is going on around you right now.

Vitality

Vitality is a human quality that exudes strength, liveliness and energy. Vitality is the ability to keep on living with zest. Vitality is the fuel of human endeavor. We are often too tired, too weak, too pooped out from are daily affairs to radiate vitality. What we eat, the fuel for the human frame, affects how we feel and think. A poor diet, lack of nutrition and healthy balance contributes to weakness, fatigue and disease. A healthy diet rich in fresh fruits and vegetables, whole grains and cereals can make us feel better. Practicing proper dietary habits is imperative to overall health and well being. You cannot exude vitality without proper nutrition. In addition to good diet, you must also have a good attitude.

Contribution

The ultimate purpose of our goals in life is to contribute something in someway to others, the world and the universe. If the purpose of your goals is self-centered and egocentric then you have missed the mark. While money and physical possessions are important they are not the sole reason for living. We should strive to make the world a little better in someway, however minor, contribute to the well being of neighbors and friends, and the world. If we have this attitude in mind when we set our goals then you will be truly successful and happy.

Summary

1. Realize how emotions can affect your health and well being.
2. Be aware of the ten negative emotions.
3. Identify which and how negative emotions affect your behavior.
4. Be aware of the ten positive emotions.
5. Focus on positive emotions to enhance your well being.

Chapter 6

Learning to Relax

We are all under a considerable amount of stress in today's world. We no longer live in the age of the traditional, rural family with a white house and picket fence. We live in a very fast paced secular society where change occurs all the time. We are exposed to minor and major stressors on a daily basis. We have incredible demands placed on ourselves. There are work and family responsibilities and commitments. Growing debt and financial strife our constant stressors. Even the daily commute to and from work or to the supermarket has become stressful. Daily, constant and unrelenting stress can have a negative effect on the human body. The effects of stress on health are well known. Chronic stress can aggravate or directly lead to illness and disease. We can show how to modify your stress response and change your reaction to stress. Follow the skills outlined here and you will have some practical stress reduction techniques that produce powerful results.

Definition

Stress is defined as any physical, mental, emotional or spiritual state that requires a response or change from a previous state. The human body has an incredible, innate capacity to maintain an internal state of balance. Homeostasis is the term used to describe this internal balance of chemicals, enzymes, metabolism and thoughts in the human body. Stress is any factor that upsets this delicate internal balance. A certain amount of stress is healthy, vital and necessary to maintain life. However, undue excessive stress upsets our natural balance and changes our internal physiology. Stress can cause wear and tear to the human body and mind. Stress can lead to illness and disease.

Symptoms of Stress

Physical response to stress by the human body include increased heart rate, increased blood pressure, increased breathing rate, tight muscles, increased perspiration, stomach tightness and clenched jaw. Psychological response to stress include inability to concentrate, poor memory, racing thoughts, inability to sit still, frustration, anger, irritability, mood swings, lack of self esteem, compelling thoughts and depression. Diseases and illness associated with stress include acne, agitation, alcohol abuse, allergies, angina, anorexia, anxiety, arthritis, asthma, autoimmune disorders, baldness, bed-wetting, bipolar disorder, bladder problems, cancer, candidiasis, canker sores, chest pains, chronic fatigue syndrome, colds, cold hands and feet, colic, colitis, constipation, costochondritis, cystitis, depression, diarrhea, emotional lability, eczema, epilepsy, fatigue, feelings of guilt, flus, flatulence, hair loss, hayfever, headaches, heartburn, heart attacks, heart palpitations, herpes, high blood pressure, hives, hypersomnia or excessive sleep, hyperthyroidism, hyperventilation, hypoglycemia or low blood sugar, hypothyroidism, inflammatory bowel disease, impotence, inability to concentrate, indigestion, infection, infertility, insomnia, irritable bowel syndrome, lack of self confidence, learning disabilities, lethargy, loss of appetite, loss of interest in normal activities, loss of pleasure, low back pain, low blood pressure, low self esteem, lupus, malaise, manic episodes, memory loss, menopause, migraines, mood swings, motion sickness, muscle aches, muscle cramps, muscle incoordination, muscle tension, nausea, neck pain, nervousness, menstrual cramps, menstrual irregularities, muscle aches, neuralgia, nightmares, obesity, overeating, pain, peptic ulcer, poor eyesight, poor immune function, poor sex drive, premenstrual syndrome, prescription drug abuse, raynaud's disease, restless leg syndrome, rheumatoid arthritis, ringing in the ears, sexual problems, shingles, skin rashes, sore throat, stomach upset, teeth grinding, tension, tiredness, trigeminal neuralgia, trouble swallowing, vertigo, vomiting and yeast infection.

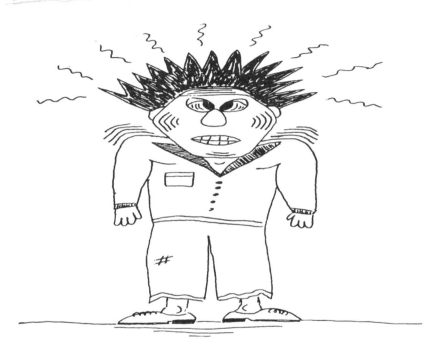

Causes of Stress

Many factors both internal and external can cause stress. Any factor that upsets the natural homeostasis in the human body can be considered a stressor. It is important to note that all stressors are not bad. The stress associated with a new job, new skill or new relationship can be considered a positive stressor. A certain amount of stress is healthy and necessary. However, negative stress can have negative effect on the human body. Major life stressors include death, birth, marriage, pregnancy, marital difficulties, financial difficulties, buying a home, mortgage problems, work problems and many other life changes. How we perceive stress is important as to it's effect on the human body.

Two individuals can be exposed to the same stressor. However, their response can differ. One individual can respond in a positive manner and benefit from the experience. The other individual can respond in a negative manner and have ill effects from the whole experience. Sometimes it is important to reframe our experiences and view them as positive, constructive stressors.

The Stress Response

The stress response involves specific physiological reactions in the human body. These effects include dilation of the pupils of the eye, the mouth dries as the salivary glands decrease production of saliva, the body starts to perspire as sweat glands are activated, the heart rate increases, blood pressure increases, the force of heart contraction increases, the bronchi in the lungs dilate, breathing becomes shallow and rapid, blood vessels constrict, digestion slows down, release of digestive enzymes ceases, stored sugar is released from the liver, the gall bladder and bile ducts relax, filtration through the kidneys slows, the bladder muscle relaxes, blood sugar levels rise rapidly, basal metabolic rate increases, adrenaline and other hormones of the adrenal glands increases, blood flow to the brain increases, mental activity increases, muscles around hair follicles in the skin become excited, blood flow to muscles increases, rapid breakdown of stored sugar occurs in muscles, muscles tense for rapid movement and muscle strength increases.

The stress response occurs in three distinct stages: the alarm stage, the resistance stage and the exhaustion stage.

Alarm Response

The first response to stress is called the alarm stage. The alarm reaction is characterized by specific physiological reactions to stress. Blood pressure and heart rate increase, breathing becomes rapid and shallow, adrenaline is released from the adrenal glands, the liver releases stored sugar, muscles tense for movement, blood flow to the digestive organs decreases, blood flow to the hands and feet decreases, blood flow to the brain and major muscles increases and the body perspires to cool itself. The main goal of the alarm reaction is to prepare the body for a quick reaction to a specific stressor. The physiological effects of the alarm reaction are primarily regulated by the hormone adrenaline. Adrenaline is a short lived hormone and the alarm reaction is a time limited acute response.

Resistance Response

The second response to stress is called the resistance stage. The resistance reaction is characterized by the body's long term reaction to chronic stress. After the initial rush of adrenaline in the alarm reaction has worn off, other hormones modulate the stress response. Cortisol and aldosterone hormones of the adrenal cortex regulate the resistance reaction. Cortisol increases the breakdown of fat, protein and stored sugar in the form of glycogen to maintain an adequate supply of sugar in the blood. Unlike fat, protein and glycogen sugar is relatively simple chemical that can be rapidly used by the body for quick energy. Aldosterone causes sodium retention in the body to help maintain proper blood pressure levels. The primary goal of the resistance reaction is to maintain the body's response to a long term, chronic stressor. However, continued and chronic stress can literally deplete adrenal gland reserves and lead to exhaustion.

Exhaustion Response

The third response to stress is called the exhaustion reaction. Continued and prolonged stress places a tremendous burden on the entire body. All organs and tissues including the adrenal glands, nervous system, brain, heart, blood vessels, liver, kidneys and immune system bear the effects of chronic stress. Specific organs and tissues can become weakened and function poorly. The effects of chronic stress manifest in different ways in different individuals. Hypoglycemia or low blood sugar often results as the regulation of proper blood sugar levels fail. The human body is designed to react to stress in acute, short bursts of the alarm and resistance reactions. Chronic, prolonged stress can literally deplete adrenal reserves and lead to exhaustion. The purpose of stress management is to elicit the relaxation response. The relaxation response is directly opposite from the stress reaction. The opposite physiological reactions occur within the human body. The heart rate slows, blood pressure slows, breathing becomes deep and relaxed, the liver stores glucose, the pupils constrict, muscles relax, blood flow to digestive organs increases, blood flow to the extremities increases, blood flow to the major muscles decreases, and blood flow to the brain and nervous system maintains at a constant level.

Natural Stress Management

Natural treatment of stress first focuses at identifying and modifying the underlying causes of stress. In many instances it is not practical advice to advise someone to simply eliminate their stressors. Instead it is important to help individuals become aware of their stressors and their stress response. Once a general awareness exists you can proceed with stress management skills.

What are the stressors in your life right now?

1. _____

2. _____

3. _____

4. _____

5. _____

6. _____

7. _____

8. _____

9. _____

10. _____

Stress Relaxation Techniques

Stress relaxation techniques are fun and easy practical skills that can help modify our stress response. These simple psychological techniques can change our view of our stressors and elicit the relaxation reaction.

Lifestyle factors play an important role in our general health and our stress response. Proper rest, daily exercise and a healthy diet are vital for optimal health. Proper rest and good sleep habits help the body rebuild and recover from stress. Poor sleep habits and insomnia can have a deleterious effect on the human body. Additionally, daily exercise is also vital for optimal health. Exercise is a great, cheap and natural stress reduction technique. A minimum of 20 minutes of aerobic exercise each day will improve your overall health and make you feel better.

The minimum prerequisites to any psychological technique in reducing stress are a quiet environment, a passive attitude and deep breathing. A quiet environment will allow you freedom from distractions and a secure place in which to practice your stress reduction exercises. A passive attitude is important to ensure your success in altering your stress response. Unabated anger and negative self thoughts are not constructive. You must be mentally and emotionally willing to practice these techniques as directed. A passive attitude will allow to free yourself from the cycle of the stress reaction. Deep breathing is the fundamental core of all stress reduction techniques. You simply cannot be relaxed if you are not breathing in an easy, deep, relaxed manner.

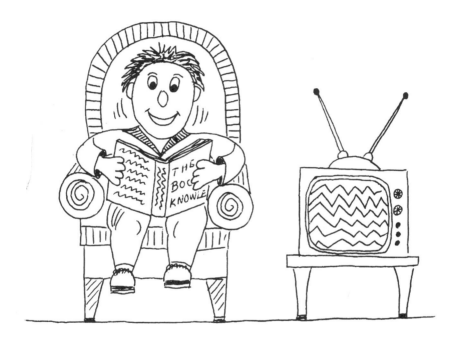

Deep Breathing

Deep, relaxed easy breathing is the cornerstone of all relaxation techniques. However, during the stress response breathing becomes rapid, laboured and shallow. Under these conditions air is forcibly inhaled and exhaled. Only the upper half of the lungs are used and the lungs never expand to their full capacity. The chest cavity rises quickly as the breathing rate is between 15 and 45 breaths per minute. Chest muscles contract rapidly for the fast, shallow breathing rate. The large diaphragm muscle separating the chest from the abdomen is not fully utilized.

During the relaxation response the breathing physiology changes. Breathing becomes slow, relaxed and deep. Under these conditions air moves in and out of the lungs passively. The entire lungs are used and the lungs expand to their full capacity. Both the chest and abdomen rise up and down with each breath. The breathing rate is between 6 and 12 breaths per minute. During deep relaxation the breathing rate seldom rises above 8 breaths per minute. With each breath the diaphragm contracts and expands into the abdomen allowing for deep, full inhalations. If you place your hand on your bellow button it will gently move up and down with each deep breath. As you breath you can feel air fill the entire lung tissue. With each deep breath you feel relaxed. Your mind relaxes as self-talk and mind chatter slows and disappears. Your muscles become less tense and relaxed. Your blood pressure and heart rate slow. Digestive muscles relax and the tightened knots in your stomach and intestines disappear.

In the relaxation response breathing is slow, relaxed and deep. The normal breathing rate at rest is between 6 and 12 breaths per minute. Each breath begins by a deep inhalation, filling the lungs with air and ends with passively exhaling and expiring air through the lungs. During the stress reaction the breathing rate is between 15 and 45 breaths per minute. Air is forcibly inhaled and exhaled as quickly as possible.

Progressive Relaxation

Progressive relaxation training is a stress reduction technique that involves tightening and relaxing groups of muscles throughout the body. The goal of progressive relaxation is to induce a state of mental and physical relaxation. By progressively tightening and then relaxing groups of muscles you can consciously control how they feel. As we physically proceed with tightening and relaxing muscle groups you also focus your mental awareness on how the muscles feel tight and how the muscles feel relaxed. Our reaction to stress often involves muscle contraction. Muscle tension can result in headaches, bruxism or teeth grinding, temporal-mandibular joint (TMJ) dysfunction, neck pain, shoulder pain, back pain, muscle spasms and other states made worse by chronic muscle contraction. Once we master the basic technique of progressive relaxation we can proceed to use this technique to help alter our stress response and induce a relaxation response in a matter of minutes. This technique is simple to use and produces dramatic and long lasting results. It must be practiced at least once per day consistently for maximum benefit. Ten different groups of muscles are used in this exercise. They are right arm; left arm; forehead; eyes, cheeks and nose; jaws, lips and tongue; neck; chest, back and shoulders; abdomen and buttocks; right leg; and left leg.

Begin by tightening all the muscles of the right arm. Tighten the fingers, the forearm and biceps and triceps muscles. Squeeze your fingers tight or make a fist. Do not move your hand or arm. Keep it firm and in one position. You may close your eyes if desired. Do not focus your attention on your breathing. Instead breath as you would normally. Contract these muscles for five to ten seconds. Focus your conscious awareness on how the right arm feels. How do the tightly contracted muscle feel at this time. After five to seconds have elapsed immediately relax the right arm. Relax all the muscles that were previously held tight. Again keep your hand in the same position as before. Do not focus your attention on your breathing. Breathe as you would normally. Focus your entire concentration on how the right arm feels. Feel how light and relaxed all the muscles feel. Keep the right arm relaxed for twenty to thirty seconds. If your mind begins to wander refocus your attention and concentration on the right arm. After twenty to thirty seconds have elapsed compare how the right arm feels when tight and contracted to how it feels when it is relaxed.

Move your attention to your left arm. Repeat the same exercise to the muscles of the left arm. Tighten and contract all the muscles of your left arm for five to seconds. After this time relax all the muscles of the left arm for twenty to thirty seconds.

Move to the forehead. Progressively tighten and relax all the muscles of the forehead. Move to the muscles around the eyes, cheeks and nose. Repeat the contraction and relaxation exercises.

Move to the muscles of the jaw, lips and tongue. Repeat the contraction and relaxation exercises to these muscles.

Move to the muscles of the neck. Repeat the contraction and relaxation exercises to these muscles.

Move to the muscles of the chest, back and shoulders. Repeat the contraction and relaxation exercises to these muscles.

Move to the muscles of the abdomen and buttocks. Repeat the contraction and relaxation exercises to these muscles.

Move to the muscles of the right leg. Repeat the contraction and relaxation exercises to these muscles.

Move to the muscles of the left leg. Repeat the contraction and relaxation exercises to these specific muscles. Notice how relaxed these muscles feel.

After you have finished moving to the different muscles groups your entire body should be relaxed. This exercise can take between seven and fifteen minutes. At the beginning it is important to practice this technique one to five times per day. As you master this technique you can employ it to alter your stress response and induce progressive relaxation to the muscles of the body.

Quieting

Quieting a simple meditation technique that quiets the mind and body. The purpose of this technique is to evoke the relaxation response and reduce tension in the brain and muscles. The technique simply involves focusing one's concentration and awareness on a special object, one's breathing or a simple word or phrase. Quieting is best carried out one or more times per day in a quiet, relaxed environment. At first you should strive to practice this technique at the same time and environment each day.

The environment should be free of distractions. You should adopt a comfortable posture, such as sitting or reclining, in which to conduct this technique. You should choose an arbitrary object, breathing or word or phrase to which you can focus your attention. Some people choose a special object such as a flower, candle or mountain stream or a word such as ohm, "one" or "love." Other people simply choose to focus their attention on their breathing technique. It is best to use only one object, word or phrase or breathing to which you focus your attention. Whatever you choose you should be comfortable with it to focus your attention for 10 to 20 minutes.

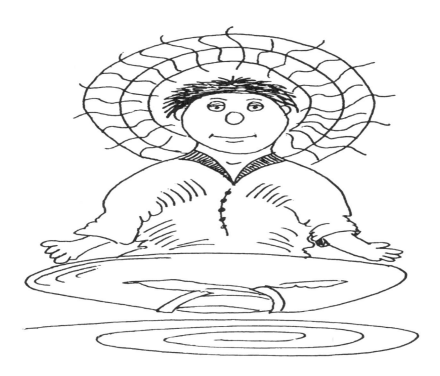

Focus on the object, repeat the word or phrase in your mind or aloud or focus on your every breath as the air moves in and out of your lungs. Your mind may begin to wander or you may be distracted at first. This is normal and you shouldn't get discouraged. When you become aware that your mind is wandering simply refocus your attention on your special object, word or phrase or breathing technique. When you first begin to practice this technique your mind may wander a lot. Don't be discouraged. Refocus your attention and concentration. You will be surprised how easy it is. Relax and enjoy this exercise. You will find you will become more relaxed and refreshed after 10 or 20 minutes.

Autogenic Training

Autogenic training is a simple relaxation technique that uses the mind to produce physical relaxation. Autogenic literally means "self-generating." This technique involves using suggestive words or phrases to generate the relaxation response. Biofeedback is a variation of this technique that uses suggestive phrases to change heart rate, blood pressure, skin conductivity and breathing rate.

By repeating suggestive phrases you can change your physiological state. You focus your attention on three physiological states: a feeling of heaviness in the body, a feeling or warmth in the body and relaxed, deep breathing. Like other relaxation techniques you should practice autogenic training in a comfortable, relaxed environment, free of distractions. You should maintain a relaxed, comfortable posture for 5 to 15 minutes. You may keep your eyes open or closed.

Begin by repeating a phrase about a feeling of heaviness in the body. Slowly repeat the phrase "my right arm is heavy" several times. As you repeat the phrase feel how heavy and weighed down your right arm actually is. After you repeat the phrase relax your right arm and now feel how light it is.

After you repeat this phrase several times repeat the phrase "my left arm is heavy." Again feel how heavy and weighed down your left arm actually feels.

Then repeat the phrase "my head is heavy."

Then repeat the phrase "my neck and shoulders are heavy."

Then repeat the phrase my back and stomach is heavy."

Then repeat the phrase "my right leg is heavy." Then repeat the phrase "my left leg is heavy."

Next repeat the entire exercise by substituting the word "warm" instead of the word "heavy." Begin by repeating the phrase "my right arm is warm." Feel how warm your arm can actually become by simply repeating this phrase. At the end of this exercise focus your attention on your breathing. In the stress response your breathing is shallow and rapid.

When you evoke the relaxation response your breathing becomes deep and slow. Do not consciously control your breathing. Just breath in a relaxed, passive manner. At the end of this exercise you will be surprised how easy it is to control your physical state at the mere repetition of a simple, suggestive phrase.

Self-Hypnosis

Self-hypnosis is a great way to induce relaxation and help you overcome your fears and problems. One patient gave me a copy of a self-hypnosis exercise that goes something like this.

1.   Identify the problem and the changes you would like to make. Say to yourself or write down: "this is what bothers me and this is what I wish would be different." Because motivation is critical as yourself: "How important is it for me to change and how committed am I to change right now?"

2. Identify the benefits
Describe to yourself the way you would like to benefit by delaying with your problem and changing the situation. List as many benefits as you can think of.

3. Imagine yourself problem-free
If you can, try to remember when you were free of your problem. How did you feel? To help you create the proper images, sit down, close your eyes and make yourself comfortable. Then imagine yourself behaving the way you want to behave, acting the way you want to act. Draw from your memory and your imagination, using all your senses. Imagine both changes and benefits. Vary colours, odours and sounds. Change, modify and play with the images until they feel right for you.

Example A.

My problem:
I get tense and anxious when I found myself in crowded places. I would like to go when and where I want to and feel relaxed.

The benefits if I change:
I'll be able to go to the theater with my friends. I'll have a wider range of jobs I can pursue. I'll be able to go with my kids to their school events. I'll feel better about myself.

The way I would like to act and feel::
I picture myself as I was at my son's fifth birthday when we went as a family to Disneyland. I felt free and easy and in love with everything, even in the midst of large crowds. I picture myself going to a Saturday matinee with my three best friends. I picture myself going to a wonderful job in the newest downtown office skyscraper.

Example B.

My Problem:
I am twenty pounds overweight and I want so much to lose weight and be slimmer at my daughter's wedding.

The benefits if I change:
I'll look better at my daughter's wedding. I'll be more photogenic for the wedding album. I'll feel better about myself. I'll be more outgoing and feel more attractive.

The way I would like to act and feel:
I picture myself going out of my way to eat what I really want. I choose from the menu very carefully, ordering exactly what I wanted. I eat very little and very slowly but savouring each and every morsel. I see myself satisfied with a lesser portion of food than usual. I see myself at my daughter's wedding looking slim and attractive, enjoying her wedding and loving the way I look and feel.

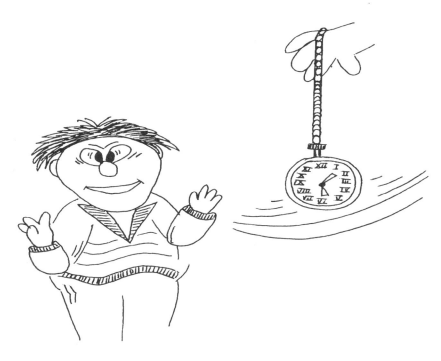

Hypnotic Induction

Get comfortable, either by sitting or lying down in a comfortable and quiet place. Make sure you will not be disturbed. Take several deep breaths all the way down to your abdomen. Close your eyes.

With your eyes closed raise them up as if you were looking at the centre of your forehead. Tell yourself that the muscles in your scalp are beginning to relax and they are letting go of all the tension. Your forehead relaxes. It becomes smooth as silk. The muscles around your eyes relax, the muscles around your mouth and cheeks let go of all the day's tension. You relax your jaw and just let it hang open. Feel the tension in your neck let go and drain away like water down the drain. Relax your shoulders and let them droop down. Let the tension flow down your arms and off your fingertips. Take another deep breath and then as you exhale let your chest relax. Relax the muscles in your back all the way down to your your tailbone. Relax the muscles in your stomach and abdomen. Let them go and let the tension fade away like a sunset. Let go of all the tension in your legs and thighs. Feel the muscles relax as the tension flows away like water down the drain. Relax the muscles of your calves, in your ankles and feet. Let the tension flow down your ankles and off your toes. Feel how relaxed your whole body feels.

See yourself stepping into an elevator. You are on the tenth floor. As the elevator starts to go down you will relax even more. Ten.... Nine.... Eight.... Relaxing deeper.... Seven.... Six.... Five.... Relaxing Deeper....Four....Three....Two....Deeper....One....Zero.

As the door of the elevator opens you find yourself on a beautiful sun-drenched beach. The beautiful Caribbean blue shimmers in the sunlight like a cut diamond. You feel the gentle warm sunshine as it shine on your face. A gentle, warm breeze blows off the water against your face. The blue water laps slowly against the sandy shoreline with a soothing rhythm. The rustle of the wind through the palm trees on the shores echoes like a soft melody. Smell the sweet aroma of palm trees, coconut and the warm Caribbean air as it wafts through your nostrils. You shiver with delight. You are even more relaxed than before. With each breath of the warm ocean you become even more invigorated than before. You have never felt this relaxed. This is paradise and you are very relaxed.

You look to your right and envision a table under some palm trees. Arranged on the table is a beautiful array of colourful tropical fruit. Drinks and delicacies of every kind. Take a moment and sample any of the fruits and drinks as you would like. Be slow and deliberate. As you reach for the fruit see the colour of banana yellow, papaya green, watermelon red and canteloupe orange. Sample as many of the fruits as you like. Smell the fruit as it approaches your face. Your mouth waters as it approaches your mouth. Your taste buds dance with delight as the fruit touches them. Taste and feel the watermelon as the juice trickles down your chin. Bite into a fresh peach or a slice of mandarin orange. Wash it down with a generous sip of lemonade, tropical fruit punch or any drink you like. Feel the fluid slide down the back of your throat.

As you indulge yourself in the tropical spread on the table, the sun begins to set against the beautiful water. Watch the sun as it bounces across the deep blue water. Watch the horizon turn from a golden yellow to a blazing orange to a fire red. Enjoy the sunset and relax yourself. This is a safe place you can come any time you want to enjoy the beauty and relax.

You are now stepping in the elevator. As the elevator begins to climb you fell your energy begin to increase as it ascend upwards. You will continue to feel totally relaxed as you did on the beach. You breathing continues to be deep, deliberate and relaxed. You feel invigorated. You feel extra confidence. One....Two....Three....Stronger....Four....Five....Six....Energized.... Seven....Eight....Nine....Alert....Ten....Recharged and refreshed.

Summary

1. Know the definition of stress.
2. Be aware of the symptoms of stress on your mind and body.
3. Be aware of the causes of stress in your life.
4. Know how your body responds to stress.
5. Practice natural stress relaxation techniques.
6. Breath deeply.
7. Practice progressive relaxation.
8. Practice quieting.
9. Practice autogenic training.
10. Practice self-hypnosis.

Chapter 7

Forgiveness and Gratitude

Forgiveness and gratitude are two of the most important nurturing and healing actions. Practicing forgiveness and showing gratitude can powerfully influence our health and well being.

Chicken Soup For Your Soul

One of the best nurturing and thought provoking books I've ever read is the simple book called "Chicken Soup For the Soul" by Jack Canfield and Mark Victor Hansen. It is a collection of different poignant stories, vignettes and poems from all walks of life. One of my favorite excerpts from the book is about one person's struggle and tribulations with suffering.

A Creed For Those Who Suffered

I asked God for strength, that I might achieve.
I was made weak, that I might learn to humbly obey...

I asked for health, that I might do great things.
I was given infirmity, that I might do better things...

I asked for riches, that I might be happy.
I was given poverty, that I might be wise...

I asked for power, that I might have the praise of men.
I was given weakness, that I might feel the need of God...

I asked for all things, that I might enjoy life.
I was given life, that I might enjoy all things...

I got nothing I asked for -- but everything I hoped for.
Almost despite myself, my unspoken prayers were answered.
I am, among men, most richly blessed.

The Buddhist philosophy recognizes that human suffering is an inevitable part of life. No one person is immune from hurt, hate, disease or some other manifestation of suffering. While some individuals unfortunately experience great suffering, all people are affected by some suffering. It is important to learn something, however small, from our trials and tribulations. Also, it is wise to count our blessings and acknowledge that life itself is a special and unique privilege. We should be forever grateful to take part in this adventure.

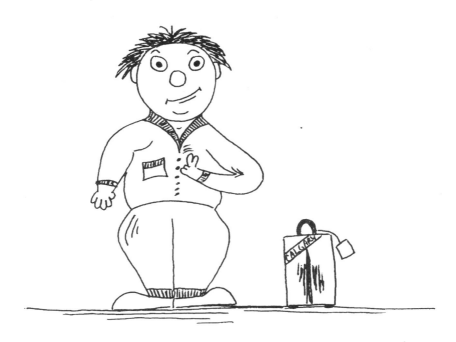

Forgiveness

Forgiveness means to pardon or excuse, on reasonable terms, one's behavior or action. Forgiveness means accepting your responsibility of your role in shaping your own life's experiences. You cannot practice forgiveness unless you start with yourself. You must acknowledge that you are doing the best you can under the given circumstances. You must accept that you are a creative power in the universe. We must forgive ourselves when we make mistakes. Disturbed human behavior is a result, in part, because people will not accept themselves as fallible and incessantly error-prone humans. Realize that you can only do the best you can and nothing more. Given all the circumstances of your life, the present situation and your current level of fitness, you are doing what you can do. In order to grow, learn, expand your horizons and find greater fulfillment in life, you must be willing to change, to take risks and try something new. By taking risks and changing you have a wonderful opportunity to practice forgiveness.

Forgiving Others

You must also forgive other people, other things and circumstances. We as humans are all fallible. Who among us hasn't made a mistake. Yes, some individuals make terrible mistakes and commit heinous crimes and should be punished for their sins. But the burden of holding and retaining our negative emotions toward their actions affects your health and well being. Anger, bitterness, depression, disappointment, discouragement, frustration, fear, guilt, hatred, hurt, loneliness, overwhelm, sadness and other negative emotions are important. They allow us to react to the circumstances in our life. They can be action calls to change are behavior, change our circumstances and change the way we think. To hold on to these negative emotions for long periods of time is unhealthy and has a negative impact on our well being. It prevents us from being happy, having inner peace and cultivating unconditional love. It prevents us from making real changes that allow us to achieve our ultimate goals. You must practice forgiveness on others to free yourself from the bondage of your negative emotions. If you want to be truly healthy then you must practice forgiveness on yourself and others around you.

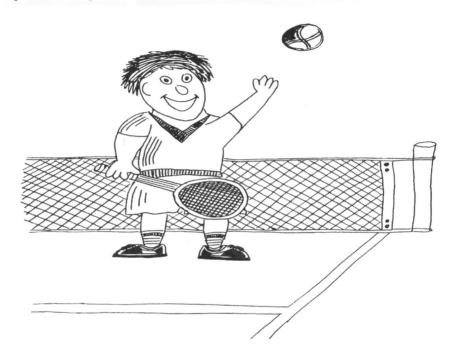

Tennis and Other Sports

Tennis and other sports are a great way to practice forgiveness. Imagine that you are playing tennis against your opponent. He serves a strong shot and you miss it. You react to the situation. You may be angry, disappointed or frustrated with yourself. You can berate yourself, scream, yell and throw your racket at the net. You can allow the missed shot to impact on the way you play the game in the future. You can upset yourself to the point of having your whole day ruined because of one missed shot. Or you can accept yourself for having missed the shot. You can feel angry, disappointed and frustrated, but just for a moment or two. You can cultivate forgiveness. You did the best you could at that time under those circumstances. You can let go of those negative emotions, learn from the situation and move on. Practicing self-forgiveness on the tennis court or in any other sport teaches us to practice self-forgiveness in other aspects of our life. On a different token, we can also be angry, frustrated and disappointed with our opponent. Again, we choose how we react to the situation. We can harbour negative emotions and affect the quality of our life in the future because of them. Or we can forgive our opponent, accept and let go. Remember, you choose your emotional reaction to the situation at hand. Cultivate forgiveness and love and you will feel better and be healthier.

Letting Go

Letting go means what it is says. It means letting go of our expectations, desires, things, ideas, thoughts, views, opinions and events. It means to stop clinging to anything and letting things unfold as they happen. It means to let go of the past, live in the present moment and stop trying to manipulate the future. It means to stop bearing grudges about past wrongs or violations. In means to stop resisting, struggling and fighting. It means to stop trying to change things except yourself. It means accepting things as they unfold. It means accepting yourself as you are. It means unconditional love. Letting go frees you of the bondage of desires and expectations. You cannot fully appreciate the present moment and cultivate mindfulness unless you practice letting go. You will free yourself of the limitations of your negative emotions. Hate, fear, anger, hurt, disappointment and guilt will melt away. You feel immediately better after you letting go and mean it.

Gratitude

Gratitude means expressing thankfulness and showing appreciation. It means to be truly grateful about one's life, circumstances, behavior and actions. It means letting go of your attachment to the negative emotions of hate, jealousy and envy. To be grateful is to show heartfelt appreciation for the simple things in life on a daily basis. Life, love and breathing are marvelous and fantastic. We should show thankfulness for our lives, our health and the incredible beauty that this world is. Practicing gratitude means to take time from our busy, frivolous lives to pay close attention to the small, heartwarming details that make our life possible.

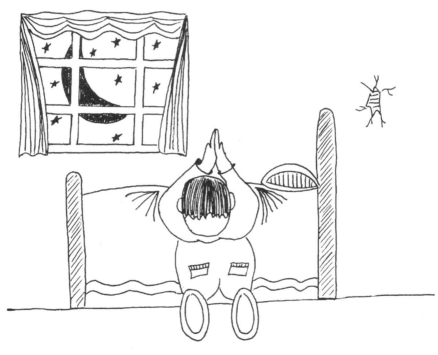

Acceptance

Acceptance of our life and circumstances means to practice forgiveness and gratitude. It doesn't mean changing your attitudes, values or beliefs. It doesn't mean having no goals or dreams. It means that we must be honest to ourselves and in the present, here and now. Some of our greatest challenges of forgiveness, gratitude and acceptance begins after we are confronted with a serious illness or disease. Bernie Siegel writes in his book "Peace, Love and Healing" about the acceptance of illness and the meaning of it.

1. Accept your illness. Being resigned to an illness can be destructive and can allow the illness to run your life, but accepting it allows energy to be freed for other things in your life.

2. See the illness as a source of growth. If you begin to grow psychologically in response to the loss of the illness has created in your life, then you don't need to have physical illness anymore.

3. View your illness as a positive redirection in your life. This means that you don't have to judge anything that happens to you. If you get fired from a job, for example, assume that you are being redirected toward something else you are supposed to be doing. Your entire life changes when you say that something is just a redirection. You are then at peace. Everything is okay and you go your own way, knowing that the new direction is the one that is intrinsically right for you. After a while you begin to feel that this is true.

4. Death or recurrence of illness is no longer seen as synonymous with failure after the aforementioned steps are accomplished, but simply as further choices and steps. If staying alive were your sole goal, you would have to be a failure because you do have to die someday. However, when you begin to accept the inevitability of death and see that you have only a limited time, you begin to realize that you might as well enjoy the present to the best of your ability.

5. Learn self-love and peace of mind and the body responds. Your body gets "live" or "energy" messages when you say "I love myself." That's no the ego talking, it's self-esteem. It's as if someone else is loving you, saying that you are a worthwhile person, believing in you and telling you that you are her to give the world something. When you do that your immune system says "this person likes living, let's fight for life."

6. Don't make physical change your sole goal. Seek peace of mind, acceptance and forgiveness. Learn to love. In the process, the disease won't be totally overlooked -- it will be seen as one of the problems you are having and perhaps one of your fears. If you learn about hope, love, acceptance, forgiveness and peace of mind, then the disease might go away in the process.

7. Achieve immortality through love. The only way you can live forever is to love somebody. Then you can really leave a gift behind. When you live that way, as many people with physical illness do, it is even possible to decide when you die. You can say, "thank you, I've used my body to the limit. I have loved as much as I possibly can and I am leaving at two o'clock today." And you go. Then maybe you have spent half an hour dying and the rest of your life living: but when these things aren't done, you might spend a lot of your life dying and only a little time living.

Summary

1. Forgive yourself for shortcomings and mistakes in life.
2. Forgive others for their shortcomings and mistakes.
2. Let go of the past mistakes, emotions and hurts.
3. Practice gratitude by being thankful and appreciative.
4. Cultivate acceptance and practice love on a daily basis

Chapter 8

The Present Moment

We are often so focused on the future, achieving our goals or so preoccupied with the past that we often forget the present moment. We can't change the past and can only prepare for an uncertain future. The only moment we can influence is the present one right now. Eventhough we all live in the present, we fail to enjoy and savour the moment to its fullest potential. And before you know it, it's gone.

What is the Present Moment?

The present moment means just that. It means paying close attention to the present moment, forgetting about the past and disregarding the future. Of course, not in a frivolous way, but rather focusing your attention to the present, how your feel and what is going on around you and how you fit in the grand scheme of things right now. One of the greatest values I've found in my limited study of eastern philosophies is their value of the present moment.

Buddha and the Moment

One of the medical doctors turned new age guru is Deepak Chopra. Once a prominent Massachusetts endocrinologist he returned to discover his ancient eastern roots in Indian philosophy. He has went on the author several bestselling books on medicine that integrates his eastern philosophy. In his books he frequently talks about the proverbs of the ancient religious deity called the Buddha. One simple, yet profound and pointed poem illustrating the transiency of our lives is taken from the Buddha.

"This existence of ours is as transient as the autumn clouds.
To watch the birth and death of beings is like looking at the movements of a dance.
A lifetime is like a flash in the sky,
Rushing by like a torrent down a steep mountain."

In the grand scheme of things our lives are very short and ethereal. Our existence is just a series of loosely related moments in time. We often tend to get philosophical about the value of our lives and those little moments, when we discuss death and dying.

Steven Levine, Death and Dying

I enjoy receiving a quarterly newsletter on midlife crises from a local counsellor who writes about the many facets of our troubled lives. In one particular newsletter he talks about the psychotherapist, Stephen Levine and his experiences with the fragility of life and death and dying. Levine has spent over twenty years accompanying the sick and ill to the threshold of death. He has found how the brink of death takes people unexpected and unaware.

"On their deathbed some people look back on their lives and are overwhelmed by a sense of failure. They have a closet full of regrets. They become disheartened when they reflect on how they have overlooked the preciousness of their relationships, forgotten the importance of finding their "true work," and delayed what some call "living my own life." Because they have left so many parts of their life for "later," they felt fragmented about unsatisfying work, unfinished business in relationships, and compromised lifestyles. But "later" came much sooner than they

expected, and they found themselves burdened by unfulfilled dreams and a sense of incompleteness."

A Terminal Prognosis

Most people do not think of death and dying. We are often too busy with work and family commitments to consider the frailty of life. Our daily schedule is full. Our lives are consumed with earning a living, meeting a deadline or arriving at a destination. Our minds are cluttered with frivolous details, facts and appointments. We often consider ourselves invincible and somehow aloof from an impending end to our short life. We fail to consider how fragile and short our existence is here on the earth. Only after we consider a terminal prognosis do we consider the meaning of our lives. A terminal prognosis means that we have a finite amount of time left here. We are going to die.

Only after a terminal prognosis is given do many people reflect upon the meaning and directions of their lives. They consider their successes and failures, hopes and dreams. They realize their shortcomings of broken promises, goals not reached and dreams not attained. Many people realize a life yet unlived. They have much more life in them and they don't want to die. After a terminal prognosis many people make dramatic changes in terms of their attitudes and direction. They may attempt things they have only dreamed about. Things that we were once important parts of their lives become seemingly trivial and unimportant. Things of lesser importance become important. They may take on a totally new and different meaning to their lives.

One Year To Live

You should attempt to live your life as if you have been given a terminal prognosis. Live as if you only had one year to live. Think about all the things you would do or change in life. Take charge of the direction your life is be going. Take responsibility for your action. Learn to act instead of react. Make an attempt to try things that you otherwise wouldn't. Strive to fulfill your dreams, however frivolous or far-fetched. Enjoy your life to the fullest.

Here and Now

Many people fail to live here and now. They are consumed by the past. Past memories clog up their mind and impair their ability to live in the present. Realize that memories are only shadows of the past. While they may be beautiful and heartwarming reflections of our past experiences, don't let them consume you and affect the present. Many people are too busy preparing or worrying about an uncertain future. Future expectations, appointments and goals consume most of their time and energies. Realize that the future is of a time yet to come. While it may be wise to prepare for the future, don't let expectations and goals consume you. Make an attempt to live in the present, here and now.

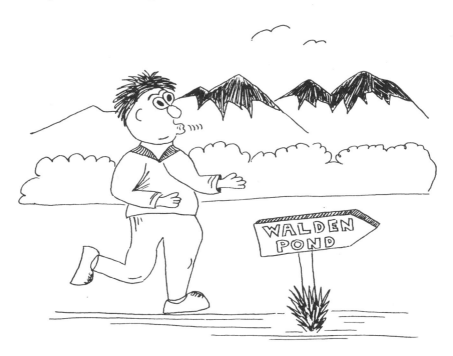

Henry David Thoreau

Henry David Thoreau was the 19th century American author who wrote the classic book "Walden." Henry was dissatisfied with his preoccupation with acquiring material possessions and his striving for acclaim in his career. He decided to build himself a one bedroom cabin on the shores of a lake called Walden Pond near Concord, Massachusetts. He lived a pleasant, meager existence there for nearly two years. The sum of what he learned there about living at it's rudimentary level is eloquently described in his book, "Walden."

The Bloom of the Present

While in his small cabin at the shores of Walden Pond, Henry David Thoreau frequently spent the entire morning sitting on his front porch observing nature around him. He literally watched the present moment develop around him

"There were times when I could not afford to sacrifice the bloom of the present moment to any work, whether of the head or hand. I love a broad margin to my life. Sometimes, in a summer morning, having taken my accustomed bath, I sat in my sunny doorway from sunrise till noon, rapt in a revelry, amidst the pines and hickories and sumachs, in undisturbed solitude and stillness, while the birds sang around or flitted noiseless throughout the house, until by the sun falling in at my west window, or the noise of some traveller's wagon on the distant highway, I was reminded of the lapse of time. I grew in those seasons like corn in the night, and they were far better than any work of the hands would have been. They were not time subtracted from my life, but so much over and above my usual allowance. I realized what the Orientals mean by contemplation and the forsaking of works. For the most part, I minded not how the hours went. The day advanced as if to light some work of mine; it was morning, and lo, now it is evening, and nothing memorable is accomplished. Instead of singing, like the birds, I silently smiled at my incessant good fortune. As the

sparrow had its trill, sitting on the hickory before my door, so I had my chuckle or suppressed warble which he might hear out of my nest."

Wherever You Go, There You Are

The clandestine practice of eastern Buddhism called mindfulness is deceitfully similar to the simple awareness of the present moment practiced by Henry Thoreau. In fact, there are one and the same. Don't be confused.

One of the easiest books I've come across on the topic of Buddhism and the practice of mindfulness in everyday life is "Wherever you go there you are" by Jon Kabat-Zinn. He does an excellent explanation of Buddhist philosophy, their understanding of the present moment and their practice of mindfulness. Remember, wherever you go, there you are. There's no escaping yourself or the present moment.

Mindfulness

Mindfulness is the ancient buddhist practice of paying close, intense, non-judgmental attention to the present moment. You don't have to be a buddhist, yogi or guru to practice mindfulness and gain its tremendous benefits. In fact, the word "buddhist" means "awakened or enlightened one." Mindfulness is a simple concept that helps to nurture greater awareness, clarity and acceptance. It is based upon the concept that our lives unfold only as moments. All we have are moments. We might as well enjoy them and gain all that we can from them. It teaches us to live in harmony with ourselves and the world around us. It is a wake up call to our consciousness.

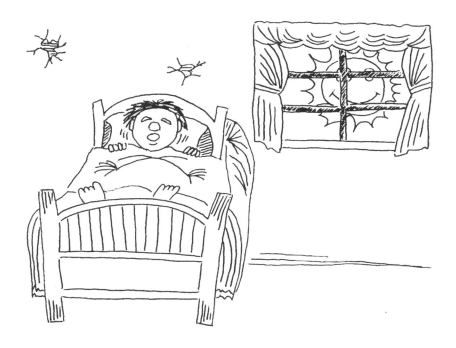

Waking Up

Our ordinary wakeful day-to-day state is blunted and dull.
Mindfulness is the practice of sharpening and waking up our
consciousness to be more aware and in tune with daily life. A
diminished awareness of the present moment creates problems for
psyche including fears, anxieties and insecurities. Mindfulness
provides a simple yet powerful route for getting ourselves unstuck
and back in tune with ourselves and the world. It is a way to take
charge of the direction and quality of our lives. It helps to nurture
our intimate relationships with ourselves and others around us. It
helps to cultivate an intense appreciation of the beauty of the world
and nature around us. It does adopt one religious outlook over
another, but can be used to heighten our spiritual relationships. It
can be used as a form of meditation or prayer. It can increase our
acceptance, clarity and awareness of god around us non-
judgmentally. It means paying close attention to the present
moment without our opinions, biases, fears, expectations or

influences. It means just paying close, intense attention to the present moment by being yourself and accepting the present moment as it unfolds before you.

The Practice of Mindfulness

Try stopping, sitting down and becoming more aware of your breathing once in while through the day. In can be for five minutes or even five seconds. Let go into full acceptance of the present moment, including how you are feeling and what you perceive to be happening around you. For these moments, don't try to change anything at all, just breath and let go. Breathe and let be. Try not to have anything be different in this moment; in your mind and in your heart, give yourself permission to allow this moment to be exactly as it is and allow yourself to be exactly as you are. Then, when you're ready, move in the direction your heart tells you to go, mindfully and with resolution.

This Is It

Two zen monks in robes and shaven heads, one young, one old, sitting side by side cross-legged on the floor. the younger one is looking somewhat quizzical and puzzled. The older monk turns to him and says "nothing happens, this is it."

"This is it." That's all there is, just the present moment. Try to just be in the present moment. Drop all your thoughts, expectations, judgments and accept the present moment. Drop all your expectations of the past and future. People usually don't get this right away. They want to meditate in order to relax, to experience a special state, to become a better person, to reduce some stress and pain, to break out of old habits and patterns, to become free and enlightened. Don't get caught up in trying to have a special experience. Just let the moment be and unfold before you. Accept it, don't judge it and you'll realize how special it actually is.   You don't have to be in a special place or an enlightened state of mind. By accepting the present moment and living in it in a conscious way you have already made it special and you have achieved enlightenment in the present moment.

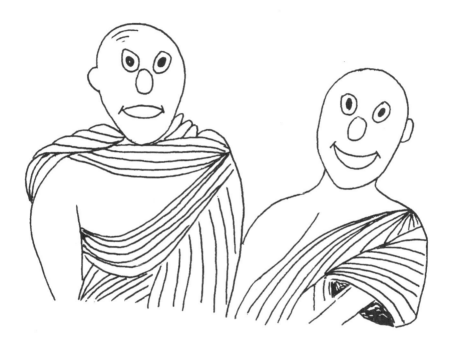

Mindfulness in the Morning

According to Henry David Thoreau, the best time to practice mindfulness is in the morning. In his book "Walden" Thoreau writes about the significance of the morning and developing a higher level of consciousness on a daily basis.

"Morning is when I am awake and there is dawn in me....We must learn to reawaken and keep ourselves awake, not by mechanical aids, but by an infinite expectation of the dawn, which does not forsake us in our soundest sleep. I know of no more encouraging fact than the unquestionable ability of man to elevate his life by conscious endeavor. It is something to be able to paint

a particular picture, or to carve a statue and so to make a few objects beautiful; but it is far more glorious to carve and paint the very atmosphere and medium through which we look....To affect the quality of the day, that is the highest of arts."

Early in the Morning

Try making a commitment to yourself to get up earlier than otherwise might. Just doing it changes your life. Awaken to the dawn of a new day and just be in the moment. You don't necessarily have to do anything. Just pay close attention to the beauty of the morning and let it unfold before you. Accept it non-judgmentally, look around and inhale its beauty. Furthermore, try pay close attention to many of the fleeting moments throughout your day. If you fail to do this you may live a life filled with many regrets.

Regret and Life to Live Over

One of the great disappointments in life is to reach old age and reminisce of a life filled with regrets. An eloquent verse taken from the book "Peace, Love and Healing" by the surgeon Bernie Seigel illustrates the conclusion of a failure to live in the present moment. An elderly lady with a terminal disease writes this prophetic verse about regrets in her life and of opportunities missed.

"If I had my life to live over, I'd try to make more mistakes next time. I would relax, I would limber up, I would be crazier than I've been on this trip. I know very few things I'd take seriously anymore. I would take more chances, I would take more trips, I would scale more mountains, I would swim more rivers and I would watch more sunsets. I would eat more ice cream and fewer beans. I would have more actual troubles and fewer imaginary ones. You see...I was one of those people who lived

prophylactically and sensibly and sanely, hour after hour and day after day. Oh, I've had my moments. And if I had it to do all over again, I'd have more of them. In fact, I'd try not to have anything else, just moments, one after another, instead of living so many years ahead of my day. I've been one of those people who never went anywhere without a thermometer, a hot water bottle, a gargle a raincoat and a parachute. If I had it to do all over again, I'd travel much lighter than I have. I would start barefoot earlier in the spring and I'd stay that way later in the fall. And I would ride more merry-go-rounds and catch more gold rings and greet more people and pick more flowers. And dance more often. If I had it to do all over again. But you see, I don't."

Summary

1. Try to live in the present moment.
2. Live your life as if you only had one year to live.
3. Appreciate the bloom of the present moment.
4. Practice the art of mindfulness.
5. Live with no regrets.
6. Try things, make mistakes and enjoy the moment.

Chapter 9

Achieving Inner Peace

We often spend our lives in a hurried, frivolous manner. We are so busy trying to achieve our goals and making a living that we forget to nurture our inner soul. It is important to reaffirm our values, attitudes and beliefs. It is useful to define our goals and exactly what it is we want. It is necessary to understand how your emotions affect you. It is wise to practice effective time management. It is vital that you take action to achieve your goals. It is healthy to relax and practice stress management. It is beneficial to live in the present moment. But to be truly happy you must have inner peace.

Secret of Inner Peace

The secret about achieving inner peace is that there is no secret. There is no one pathway, no one religion, no one guru that can direct or impart inner peace on everyone. Achieving inner peace is a very real, personal and individualistic experience. You don't suddenly or magically get there, wherever that is and are fully enlightened. It is an ongoing process or struggle that takes our entire lifetime to achieve. You work at it all the time. I can only offer you some direction and enlightenment about the pathway you choose in achieving inner peace.

Finding Inner Peace

All people search for elusive inner peace. However, most people search for inner peace outside themselves. The American author Ralph Waldo Emerson said it best in his essay Self Reliance, *"People measure their esteem of each other by what each has, and not by what each is....Nothing can bring you peace but yourself."* The ancient Greek philosopher Marus Aurelius was quoted as saying, *"No where can a man find a quieter or more untroubled retreat than his own soul."* You can only find inner peace within yourself.

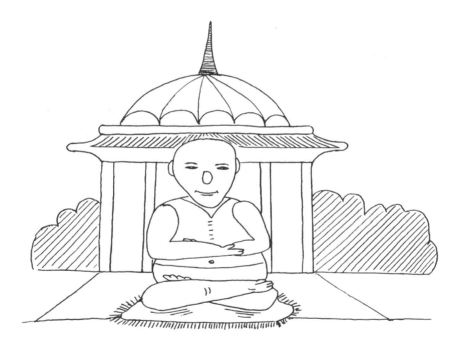

Achieving Inner Peace?

The therapist Abraham Maslow eloquently said that each person must find their own pathway to achieve inner peace; "A musician must make music, an artist must paint, a poet must write, if he is to be ultimately at peace with himself." Nobody can tell you what to do to achieve inner peace. You yourself must find out what it is you must do to achieve inner peace.

Pathways to Health

One of the best book I've ever read on health problems is called the "Sinus Survival" by Robert S. Ivker, an osteopathic doctor from Colorado. He shows that achieving good health is imperative in overcoming chronic sinusitis. He further illustrates the connection between good health and inner peace.

Part of the pathway in achieving inner peace is good health. If you can make the commitment to give yourself just over an hour a day to practice good health, I can assure you it will make a profound difference in the quality of your life. You will soon understand that health is much more than just the absence of physical disease. As you gain heightened awareness of your health you will be on your road to achieving inner peace.

- You will be more present with whatever it is you're doing.
- Experience a greater level of physical fitness.
- Let go of your ego and old, conditioned behavior patterns.
- Take more risks.
- Be more child-like and have more fun.
- Be more accepting of pain.
- Listen to your intuition and make better choices.
- Spend more time with supportive people.
- Be better able to give others as well as to receive.
- See your life as a mirror reflecting back to you your unconscious thoughts and feelings.
- Respect and better appreciate your home, the earth and all its inhabitants.
- Trust and have more faith and much less fear.
- Recognize that all of your dreams can become a reality.
- Realize anything is possible.
- Live while you're alive.

Your personal health is important in your quest to attain inner peace. While your physical well being is consuming, your emotional, mental and spiritual health is as as important. As you improve all aspects of your personal health you will experience symptoms of inner peace.

Bernie Siegel, Love and Healing

Bernie Siegel is the dynamic American surgeon who has written several bestselling books including "Love, Medicine and Miracles" and "Peace, Love and Healing." He integrates his hard core medical philosophy with the compassion and warmth that only a gifted healer can have. I think these books should be standard reading for all cancer patients and those with chronic debilitating disease. He writes and talks in every day language that is easy to understand and comprehend. He writes with much wit, wisdom and humour that we can relate to and integrate into our daily lives. From his book, "Peace, Love and Healing", there is a list of the symptoms of inner peace.

Symptoms of Inner Peace

In our fast paced, busy, secular lives it is often too easy to get cluttered with information overload and lose touch with our inner self. We should take time each day to meditate and reflect on achieving inner peace. By practicing these symptoms of inner peace you will improve your health and well being.

- Tendency to think and act spontaneously rather than from fears based on past experiences.
- An unmistakable ability to enjoy each moment.
- Loss of interest in judging self.
- Loss of interest in judging other people.
- Loss of interest in conflict.
- Loss of interest in interpreting actions of others.

- Loss of ability to worry (this is a very serious symptom).
- Frequent, overwhelming episodes of appreciation.
- Contented feelings of connectedness with others and nature.
- Frequent attacks of smiling through the eyes of the heart.
- Increasing susceptibility to love extended by others as well as the uncontrollable urge to extend it.
- Increasing tendency to let things happen, rather than make things happen.

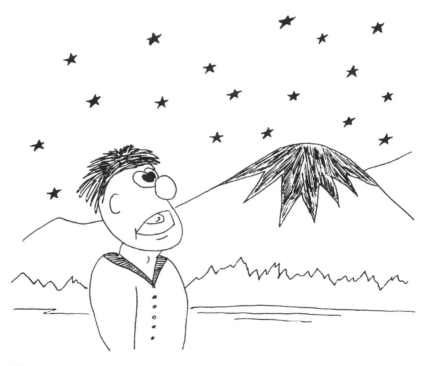

Life Satisfaction

In his book, "Ageless Body, Timeless Mind" Deepak Chopra outlines and explores the various factors that influence aging in the human body. Many of these factors that influence aging also promote disease and degeneration. He discusses the importance of life satisfaction as a prevention for disease and aging. One of the important aspects of inner peace is life satisfaction. You must derive daily satisfaction and some meaning from your life.

- Take pleasure from daily activities.
- Regard your life as meaningful.
- Achieve your major goals.
- Hold a positive self-image.
- Be optimistic.

A Different Drummer

The 19th century American author Henry David Thoreau wrote that each individual should march the beat of their own drummer, avoid competing with others to measure your success and avoid the trap of acquiring material possessions. Instead he emphasized that we should focus our attention on our inner sanctum and the development of our soul.

"Why should we be in such desperate haste to succeed and in such desperate enterprises? If a man does not keep pace with his companions perhaps it is because he hears a different drummer. Let him step to the music he hears, however measured or far away. It is not important that he should mature as soon as an apple tree or oak. However mean your life is, meet it and live it; do not shun it and call it hard names. It is not so bad as you are. It looks poorest when you are richest. The fault-finder will find faults even in paradise. Love your life, poor as it is. You may perhaps have some pleasant, thrilling, glorious hours, even in a poorhouse. The setting sun is reflected from the windows of the almshouse as brightly as from the rich man's abode. Cultivate poverty like a garden herb like sage. Do not trouble yourself much to get new things, whether clothes or friends. Turn the old; return to them. Things do not change; we change. Sell your clothes and keep your thoughts. God will see that you do not want society. It is life near the bone where it is sweetest. Superfluous wealth can buy superfluities only. Money is not required to buy one necessary of the soul."

Characteristics of Longevity

Quality of life is as important as quantity of life. Some of the most long lived people often exhibit exuberance and happiness in daily life. In his book "Ageless Body, Timeless Mind" Deepak Chopra explores the important characteristics of longevity. These include:

- Having a stable family life.
- Regarding their marriages as satisfying.
- Rarely living alone.
- Continuing to grow in their careers.
- Having no disabling mental illness.
- Not being an alcoholic.
- Having fewer chronic illness.

If you want to achieve longevity you should practice and should try to develop these characteristics. However, it should be pointed out that sometimes you have no control over some of these extraneous factors

How to Live to a 100

In his book "Ageless Body, Timeless Mind" Deepak Chopra further explores longevity. He provides some habits that are conducive with long life. Some of the characteristics traits of those individuals who live to a 100 years old or more are:

- Eat frugally.
- Get plenty of fresh air.
- Exercise daily.
- Choose a congenial occupation.
- Develop a placid, easy-going personality.
- Maintain a high level of personal hygiene.
- Drink wholesome liquids.
- Abstain from stimulants and sedatives.
- Get plenty of rest.

- Have a bowel movement once per day.
- Live in a temperate climate.
- Enjoy a reasonable sex life.
- Get proper medical attention when needed.

Ten Keys to Active Mastery

In his book, "Ageless Body, Timeless Mind" Deepak Chopra outlines ten keys to active mastery in life. Like any skill these essential keys must be practiced daily for best results.

- Listen to your body's wisdom.
- Live in the present, for it is the only moment you have.
- Take time to be silent, to meditate, to quiet the internal dialogue.
- Relinquish the need for approval.
- When you react with anger or opposition, realize you are only struggling against yourself.
- Know that the world "out there" reflects your reality in here.
- Shed the burden of judgment -- you will feel much lighter.
- Don't contaminate your body with toxins, with junk food, drink or toxic emotions.
- Replace fear-motivated behavior with love-motivated behavior.
- Understand that the physical world is just a mirror of a deeper intelligence.

Life is a creative enterprise. There are many levels of creation and therefore, many levels of possible mastery. To be completely loving, nonjudgmental and self-accepting is an exalted goal, but the important things is to work from a concept of wholeness. Because society lacks a vision of the road's end, the eminent psychiatrist Erik Erikson laments, *"Our civilization does not really harbor a concept of the whole of life."* The new paradigm provides us with such a concept, knitting body, mind and spirit into unity. The later years should be a time when life becomes whole. The circle closes and life's purpose is fulfilled. In that regard, active mastery is not just a way to survive to extreme old age -- it is the road to freedom.

Faith

Faith is an unwavering confidence or trust in yourself or another person. Faith most commonly refers to a belief in god, a higher power or a distinct religious system. Faith was once considered a belief in something without scientific proof. Prayer is one way to practice faith.

A fascinating study conducted by a cardiologist researched whether or not prayer would affect the health of heart patients at a busy San Francisco Hospital. The patients were assigned to different groups. One group were regularly prayed for and one group was not prayed for at all. The patients, staff and doctors were unaware as to which group they were assigned. The patients who were regularly prayed for had significantly fewer life threatening events and complications during their stay at the hospital. This is a fascinating study that implies that prayer and faith can influence the outcome of disease processes. Ofcourse further study is needed to elaborate on the validity of this. The ramifications of studies like this is tantamount. Don't wait till the scientific community validates the power of faith. Practice faith in yourself, others and your higher power on a daily basis. The old proverb say it best, *"With faith, you can move mountains."* You should strive to practice faith about yourself and your higher power, whomever and whatever that is.

Hope

Hope is a feeling of confidence in that the future will turn out. It is a desire that accompanies expectation and anticipation. Hope embodies a positive attitude and a feeling of optimism. We all have hopes and dreams about ourselves, friends, families and the world. Through ill health, sickness, circumstances or by choice our feeling of hope becomes dull and blunted. Yes, there are many bad, unspeakable horrors and grave injustices that happen throughout the world. Bad experiences befall us all and frequently leave a bad taste in our mouth. However, there is still some good in the world. There are good, decent people everywhere. There are good events and charitable actions, however small and seemingly insignificant. You must strive to practice hope and optimism and work at having a good attitude. When you are hopeful you create a compelling future for yourself and others.

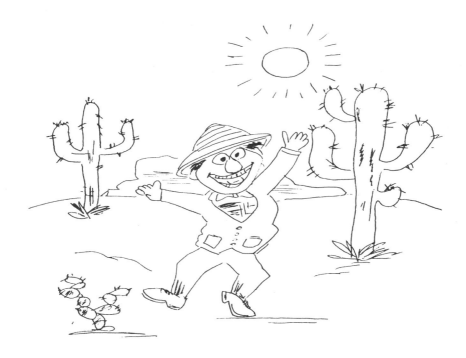

Success

One of the best quotations of the meaning of success was by the 18th century American essayist, philosopher and clergyman, Ralph Waldo Emerson.

"To laugh often and much; to win the respect of intelligent people and the affection of children; to earn the appreciation of honest critics and endure the betrayal of false friends; to appreciate beauty, to find the best in others; to leave the world a bit better, whether by a healthy child, a garden patch or a redeemed social condition; to know even one life has breathed easier because you have lived. This is to have succeeded."

Personal Mission Statement Restated

The most effective way I know about ending this little journey is the write a personal mission statement. A personal mission statement is a creed to live by. It is a brief summarizing statement about your set of principles or opinions. It outlines your most important values, attitudes and beliefs. It focuses on your achievements and goals. It defines your personal character, who you want to be and your contributions you want to make. Define the type of person you want to be, write down your own personal mission statement.

_____

_____

_____

_____

_____

_____

_____

The final step in reaching your goals and achieving inner peace is to be the type of person you outlined in your personal mission statement. Strive to be that person each and every day.

Summary

1. Realize only you alone can achieve inner peace.
2. Follow the pathway to inner peace.
3. Exhibit the symptoms of inner peace.
4. Derive life satisfaction.
5. March to the beat of a different drummer, if necessary.
6. Be aware of the characteristics of longevity.
7. Follow the prescription for a long, fruitful life.
8. Practice the ten keys of active mastery.
9. Strive for faith and hope.
10. Succeed on your own terms.
11. Have a firm personal mission statement.

Index

Suggested Reading List

Butler, Gillian and Hope, Tony: *Managing Your Mind,* Oxford University Press, New York, NY, 1996.

Canfield, Jack and Hansen, Mark Victor: *Chicken Soup For The Soul*, Health Communications, Inc. Deerfield Beach, Florida, 1993.

Chopra, Deepak: *Ageless Body, Timeless Mind*, Harmony Books, Random House,New York, NY, 1984.

Chopra, Deepak: *Creating Health*, Houghton Mifflin Company, New York, NY, 1987.

Covey, Stephen R. : *The Seven Habits of Highly Effective People*, Simon & Schuster,New York, NY, 1990.

Cousins, Norman: *Anatomy of An Illness*, Bantam Books, New York, NY, 1997.

Frank, Viktor E. : *Man's Search For Meaning*, Washington Square Press, Simon & Schuster, New York, NY, 1984.

Gallwey, Timothy W. : *Inner Tennis*, Random House, New York, NY, 1976.

Ivker, Robert: *Sinus Survival*, G. P. Putnum's Sons, New York, NY, 1988.

Kabat-Zinn, Jon: *Wherever You Go There You Are*, Hyperion Books, New York, NY, 1994.

Robbins, Anthony: *Awaken The Giant Within*, Simon & Schuster, (A Fireside Book), New York, NY, 1994.

Robbins, Anthony: *Unlimited Power*, Fawcett Columbine Books, Ballantine Books, New York, NY, 1986.

Siegel, Bernie S. : *Peace, Love and Healing*, Harper & Row Inc., New York, NY, 1990.

Suzuki, David: *Inventing The Future*, Stoddart Publishing Company, Toronto, Canada, 1989.